Full Heart Empty Womb

How I survived Infertility ... Twice

Stephanie A Greer
Jeremiah 29:11

By

Stephanie Greer

Full Heart Empty Womb

© 2014 Copyright Stephanie Greer

ALL RIGHTS RESERVED. No part of this document may be reproduced or transmitted in any form whatsoever, electronic, or mechanical, including photocopying, recording, or by any informational storage or retrieval system without express written, dated and signed permission from the author, except for the inclusion of brief quotations in a review or article, when credit to the book and order information are included in the review or article.

Full Heart Empty Womb

Dedication

To my family. This is our Love story.

Full Heart Empty Womb

Table of Contents

Chapter 1 – Boy Meets Girl..................................1

Chapter 2 – My Big Orange Binder.........................8

Chapter 3 – A Very Bumpy Road........................26

Chapter 4 – Highs & Lows..................................50

Chapter 5 – Miracle High....................................66

Chapter 6 – A Change of Heart...........................84

Chapter 7 – My Unique Grief.............................127

Chapter 8 – A Little Monday Quarterbacking..........134

Chapter 9 – In Eric's Own Words.......................153

Chapter 10 – In Her Own Words........................ 160

Full Heart Empty Womb

Foreword

When I heard that my friend, Stephanie, was planning to write this book I eagerly offered to edit it for her. I met Stephanie in 2006 as a fellow passenger on the infertility rollercoaster. I (along with my husband) met Stephanie and Eric in a couple's infertility support group at a local adoption agency – just the way we all want to make friends, right? Perhaps even more significant is the fact that we were the only two couples in the group! I knew when we met them that we would be good friends. We could meet each other in a vulnerable place that would give us a unique opportunity to be present for someone else that was going through the exact same grief and turmoil that we were. Until we met someone else going through infertility, we had felt completely alone in our experience. Because the support of other women and couples struggling with infertility was the single biggest comfort and source of hope during my journey to motherhood, I wanted to be a part of Stephanie's effort to help others cope with the many ups and downs of infertility. The minute I saw her big, orange binder (you'll laugh out loud when you read about it!), I knew this woman had a heart and determination that I wanted to absorb while going through infertility alongside her. Sometimes I just wanted to give in to hopelessness. Stephanie wanted to give infertility a roundhouse kick. And she did. But what Stephanie imparts to us in her book is that we ALL give infertility a roundhouse kick every time we cry, shake it off, and move on to the next test or cycle or procedure. What Stephanie gives is hope and strength for the journey. The outcome may not always be quick, painless or positive. But we can become stronger, more connected to our inner self, more spiritual, and even more *hopeful* as we face disappointment and perhaps the hardest journey many of us will experience in our lifetime. Happily, Stephanie's experience included success in conception and birth. But I think she would say after her second journey through infertility (and a not-so-happy outcome) that the greatest gift she received along the way was acceptance. How did she do it? How did she gain acceptance? Enjoy her words of wisdom and encouragement here. Be prepared to cry, relate, cheer her on, and even laugh out loud. If you can't imagine anything funny about infertility, read on. I believe by the end of the book you will feel more empowered and hopeful and most importantly, less alone. I wish much peace to you.

Rachael R. Hamilton

Tampa, FL

Chapter One – Boy Meets Girl

Spring 2005

Another night with a tear streaked pillow. My hair is matted to my face where the tears have soaked my brown hair. I have given up even wiping them because they are flowing so fast. Occasionally a sob will erupt from my lips. I clutch my belly. Half a prayer and half just to myself I cry, "Why can't I be normal? When will it be my turn?"

Eric lays a supportive hand on my back. I can tell he wants to say something but is at a loss for words. So he just rubs my back and tells me he loves me and our day will come. This goes on for hours. Eric's hand stays on my back but goes limp. My tears slow until they are just all cried out. Eventually exhaustion wins the night's battle and I fall into a restless sleep.

I wake up the next morning with my eyes swollen from the night before. I shower and dab some eye cream on my tired eyes in hopes that it will help them feel just a little better. Eric looks at me and I can tell he wants to say something but just doesn't know what to say. He kisses my head, rubs my back and tells me to have a good day. He assures me that today will be better and suggests that we go on a date this weekend.

I trudge down to my office wishing I was a coffee drinker. Surely a jolt from a cup of joe would improve my morning. I fire up my email ready to start my day at work. I see a string of emails from girlfriends. Apparently I am the last to see it. The subject line: "Guess who is expecting??" And I am pulled right back under. I have never been so thankful for my home office as the sobs overtake my body again.

Full Heart Empty Womb

January 1998 – University of Tennessee

Statistics class in college. At respectable dinner parties that is where I tell people I met my husband, Eric. It is what I hoped to tell my someday, maybe, hopefully, pretty please God, future children. That isn't a total lie. We were in statistics class together but our first meeting was quite different.

Football season was over so the normal barrage of parties had died down. After a month at home with our families for Christmas and an intense start of the spring semester, my girlfriends and I were excited for a Saturday night of band parties on fraternity row. It was one of those nights that you look back on ten years later and think, "That is what college was all about."

Always the planner, I was talking to my girlfriends and trying to figure out which houses we wanted to go to and the order in which we would hit them. That was when Marguerite spoke up about making sure we hit the KA house before the night was over. Word on the street was that late at night they would strip and go tarp sliding in the back yard. Hello? How could we pass that up? Tarp sliding sounded like so much fun. Add into that some naked co-eds? Slam dunk for the evening! There also happened to be a cute KA that I often saw around campus.

Our first and only stop that night would be where I met my future husband. We got our off-brand red cups and went straight for the keg. There was a great 80s cover band playing so we were in heaven.

And then there he was. KA t-shirt guy. Tall, dark, and handsome. I tried to will him to look at me. Please, please look at me. Another song came on and I got the sense that someone who smelled very good was right behind me. KA t-shirt guy? Nope. He was still across the way completely oblivious of Steph. My friends nodded in another direction, gave me an encouraging look and mouthed, "*He's* cute!"

I turned around and looked up into the most beautiful pair of green eyes I have ever seen. He smiled and I was gone. An adorable dimple appeared and his smile went straight up to his eyes. I never understood how *eyes* could smile until I saw him. Those eyes went from beautiful to amazing.

The rest of the night was a blur. I quickly fell head over heels for this guy named Eric. I learned Eric was from the same hometown as my friend, Sherrell, and also happened to be in my Statistics class.

Until now, Statistics class had been a means to an end. But now…now I was absolutely giddy about going to Statistics class. 10:10 couldn't get here quickly enough. I actually showered and got dressed for class! No ball cap. No Nike pants and sweatshirt. I was dressed to impress.

We dated until I graduated from the University of Tennessee a year before him. We dated long distance for two years while he pursued his Masters in Accounting. I moved to Louisville, Kentucky where I got a job in sales with General Electric.

It was tough having a long distance relationship. Especially since he, like most males, isn't the best communicator. Back then it wasn't as easy to communicate as it is now. He didn't have a cell phone. There was no texting. I had an email through work but he didn't email that much. Don't even get me started on the old fashioned letters that I hinted for but never got! We were pretty much left with the telephone that he shared with four other guys in the house in which he lived. But we knew we were meant to be together and God watched over our relationship.

The Greers, Established 2002

In August of 2002 we got married and settled in Nashville, Tennessee. I didn't think I could be any happier. We had our whole life ahead of us. We both had a good start to our careers. We were happy and madly in love. We spent every weekend trying to make our house a home. And if we weren't at a football game, we were at a wedding. We were at the age that all of our friends were getting married. And since we lived in the heart of the Southeastern Conference, one didn't get married on a game weekend! We went on dates and fun trips when we could afford it. It truly was the honeymoon period.

My maternal side emerged after only a few months and I begged to get a puppy. After little persuasion, I convinced Eric to let us get Majors (named after famed UT football coach, Johnny Majors). He was my baby.

As I mentioned before, I am a planner. When I first started with GE, I went into a Franklin Covey store and spent my paycheck on a beautiful planner. A planner that could not only help me plan my day in A, B, and C order, but I could plan six months ahead - even two years ahead! It served me well in my career. I planned meetings. I planned contests for my sales team. I planned trainings. I made plans about plans. I always had a plan and that kept me sane in a stressful, high demand workplace.

I also had a plan for the Greers. Get married. Enjoy being newlyweds for two years. Have our first child. Wait another couple of years and have our second. If we have two kids that are the same gender, then try for a third in another two years. It would be that simple, right? For some, maybe so.

It took a little more convincing than I anticipated to get Eric on my plan's timeline. But after much campaigning, I got him on my timetable. I couldn't help it. I was so ready to become a mother. All my life I have loved kids. I made all my money in high school babysitting the kids in my neighborhood. I never had a lot of clarity on what my career would be but I always knew I would be a mother. And I was ready now.

One of my good friends, Kristin, was a great resource to me. She had already had her first child. She was a nurse and she loved to help people. I wanted to know everything I needed to know about how to get pregnant and she was ready and willing to help.

I learned about tracking my temperatures to figure out when I was ovulating. I learned what ovulation is and why it is so important. She told me when we should and shouldn't try. She even shared with me some old wives' tales like how long I needed to stay lying down so the sperm could do their job. We were going to hit the ground running. I was so excited. I just knew that we were going to start trying and instantly get pregnant.

It was exciting at first. When I told Eric we had to have sex every other day, he wondered why we hadn't started trying sooner! I lingered in the baby aisle at Target. Need this. Need this. Must have this!! Oh I can't wait to register! I passed through the maternity section and imagined my growing belly in the different outfits. I calculated due dates. I imagined clever ways to announce my pregnancy. I even picked up the book, "What to Expect When You are Expecting." Can't be too prepared!

Our first attempt to conceive coincided with a trip to New York City for Thanksgiving. I didn't even have a glass of wine because I was SURE that I was pregnant. Granted, the sperm hadn't even had a chance to fertilize the egg, but I just KNEW I was pregnant and wasn't going to take a chance.

Diagnosis: Infertile

That is the way it was for a couple of months. Then my obsessive nature took over. I started not only checking my basal body temperatures each morning, but I put the results in an Excel spreadsheet and even made a graph! As silly as it was it gave me the first indication that I was INFERTILE. As I looked at my temperatures it became clear that I wasn't ovulating until very late. I didn't ovulate until day 28 and my cycle was only 34 days long.

Being a take charge kind of gal, I made an appointment with my OBGYN. I went in armed with my graphs so we could figure out what to do. I went through a battery of blood tests to figure out what was going on with me. I will always be grateful to my doctor for listening to me. Traditionally you have to try unsuccessfully to conceive for 12 months (a full year!) before you are given a workup and treatment for infertility. We had only been trying to get pregnant for a few months. But it was quite clear that my body wasn't doing what it needed to do for us to get pregnant.

I was so frustrated. Something was *wrong* with me. Why can't my body do what it is supposed to do? I mean, I *am* a woman, right? Had I done something to cause this? Was I just getting what I deserved? I did have a little wild phase in college. Why couldn't I just be normal? *Everyone* was getting pregnant around me! No problem at all. They just went off the pill and poof! They were pregnant. And then there were those who weren't even trying that were getting pregnant too! I felt like a failure. And it didn't seem to bother Eric that much and that made me mad. He didn't understand why I was so upset.

The blood tests confirmed everything that my temperatures indicated. I needed help to get me to ovulate on time. According to my doctor, I needed to take Clomid® to help me ovulate more regularly. I also needed to take progesterone after I ovulated. I had what is called a Luteal Phase Defect which means that the time between ovulation and the start of my next cycle isn't long enough. My uterine lining would shed before an embryo even had enough time to implant. The progesterone would prolong the luteal phase (keeping my uterine lining intact) so that if I got pregnant the embryo would have enough time to implant.

It felt good to have a plan. My OBGYN said she would let me cycle like this for a few months but after that she would refer me to a reproductive endocrinologist (RE) for further evaluation. That was fine by me because I was going to get pregnant the first month. If not the first, then certainly the second! She also wanted Eric to go to an urologist to be evaluated as well. This proved to be a vital step in our diagnosis.

So that brings us back to me sitting in my office chair after getting another pregnancy announcement email. Bawling my eyes out and hugging Majors, my fur baby, for dear life. I went from a life that was living wedding shower to wedding ceremony of all my friends to a life of weekly pregnancy announcements and baby showers. That is where we were in life. A time when even a simple question like "Guess what?" got an excited "You're pregnant!!!!" in return. No…I just found a good pair of jeans. While all of my other friends in their mid to late 20s were deciding to just "go off birth control and see what happens," I was taking drugs just to give me a prayer of conceiving.

Little did I know that this would be a nearly ten-year journey for us. It would be a journey that would bring me a lot of tears but even more strength. A journey that against all odds brought me closer to my husband and taught me that I had to trust and lean on God. Through much of the journey I felt like I was all alone. Unless you have been through infertility, you just cannot understand how isolated it makes you feel. I have many reasons for writing this book. The first and foremost one is this: YOU ARE NOT ALONE. Please join me on my journey. If you are infertile, I think you will be able to identify with some of it. Hopefully that will help you to know that you aren't the only one who feels this way. If you happen to have a loved one who is struggling to conceive, perhaps this will give you a small glimpse into the trials and agony of infertility.

Chapter Two – My Big Orange Binder

Clomid® Hell

I remember picking up my first Clomid® prescription and being *excited*. "This is it!!" I thought. The answer to all of our problems! This little miracle pill is going to make my body do what it is supposed to do. Hooray!

You know that little list of possible side effects that you throw away after you get your meds? Yeah. Those are pretty important. It didn't take many doses for me to realize that Clomid® is, in fact, the devil in a small pill. Clomid® isn't for sissies. You are supposed to take it each day around the same time. I would stare at the clock to see when it was time so I wouldn't miss it by a minute.

I completely underestimated the hot flashes that are a side effect. I would wake up each night at 2:14 hot and sweaty. My legs in particular would feel like they were on *fire*. I would throw covers off of me. If I hadn't already turned the AC down, I would sneak downstairs and crank it down. Then I would turn the ceiling fan on high. After I stripped down, I would lay on top of the covers and pray for sleep. And heaven help Eric if he even thought about rolling over to my side of the bed. "NO!!!! I am too hot!!" Instead the poor thing would be curled up in the fetal position shaking because he was so cold. I had a whole new respect for my mom and menopause!

So now I am sad because I am infertile. Stressed about the drugs and getting everything right. Tired because I can't sleep at night because my body turns into Mount Kilauea at 2:14 every night. Add to that the fact that Clomid® can also make you more emotional. Fabulous. As if you even needed a reason to be emotional on top of everything else. Now you are adding a hormone that multiplies it all!

I remember one day I had a meeting out of the office when I was supposed to take my dose of Clomid®. I realized halfway there that I had forgotten to bring it with me. I drove hysterically back home to get it. I was so scared that taking it ten minutes late was going to ruin my whole cycle. Then the whole month would be a waste and we would have to wait until the next month. We put so much intense pressure on ourselves. Was taking Clomid® ten minutes or even an hour late going to prevent me from being able to get pregnant? I certainly thought it was. Looking back it was kind of arrogant to think that it was everything that Stephanie was doing that was going to get me pregnant. In reality it never was in my hands at all. Did I need to be a responsible patient? Absolutely. I definitely needed to follow the doctor's orders and instructions to the best of my ability. However if it was within just my control of getting pregnant, wouldn't I be pregnant already?

Male Factor

We went through four cycles on Clomid®. Each cycle I just knew that this was the one in which I would get pregnant. During the fourth one Eric was finally able to see his urologist. We found out that he had several really small varicoceles that affected his sperm motility. He had little to no motility. Instead of his sperm racing straight to the egg they just sort of ran around in circles. As devastating as it was, we had a little laugh about it. Eric is a very laid back person. In the morning he pours his coffee and just pokes around the house for an hour. When we are trying to get out of the house, he meanders around gathering this and that to bring along. Apparently his sperm took after him!

Ideally when you get a diagnosis you get a clear answer about what to do next. Take this medicine. Have this surgery. Change your diet. Exercise. That wasn't at all the case with us. We weren't sure what caused it. Being in a hot tub could cause the lack in motility. Of course we had just been on a trip and Eric loves a good soak in a hot tub before bed. If that were the case, then they could return to normal

Full Heart Empty Womb

in a few months. Eric had also been diagnosed with high blood pressure. Could that be why? Was it the varicoceles? They were so small that they were inoperable. We could try but it wasn't very likely they could even be repaired. It was frustrating. We certainly didn't want him to have surgery if we didn't even know for sure if that would fix our problems. Then we still had my issues with which to contend.

It was a couple of days before I could take a home pregnancy test during my fourth Clomid® cycle. I remember it well since we had taken the day off because we were about to close on a house we had just finished building. We were sitting in our favorite Mexican restaurant just giddy about our new home. We just knew that I was pregnant. I had never had such a long cycle, so we were sure that the Clomid® and Progesterone had done the trick in spite of our sperm issues. Mentally I had already decorated the room that would be the perfect nursery. All I needed to know now was if we needed to paint it pink or blue! I felt that sharp pain in my lower belly and knew our hopes and dreams were postponed again.

After calling my OBGYN, she had me come in for another round of blood tests. I dropped everything and rushed to her office and barely made the closing on our house. That is one of the many hard things about infertility. You are at the complete mercy to your cycle days and tests. It doesn't matter if you have something else that you have to do. If it is a cycle day on which you have to have a blood test or ultrasound, then you have to do it. The next day your hormone levels will be different and that may make all the difference in your diagnosis. And heaven forbid it land on a weekend and your doctor doesn't have another lab you can go to instead. It can completely throw off your entire cycle!

I think that is something that people who don't live with infertility don't understand. You have no control over anything. Your body isn't working the way it is supposed to. You can't plan anything because you never know when you have to go to the doctor. You are living day to day based on what your body does or doesn't do. You never know when you may have to go have a blood test or an ultrasound. You can't do it when it fits into your schedule. You go when you are told or you miss the boat for your cycle. Your cycle may be a month; or in some cases it feels like it lasts forever! That was usually the case for me. A few times I even had to take a drug to make me start my period because it was taking so long. People who don't understand infertility think, "So what is another month or so?" Another month is everything when your life is consumed with your infertility. It feels like an eternity.

After visiting with my OBGYN we decided it was time to move on to the next step. She gave me recommendations for a couple of fertility clinics in Nashville. Of course it took time to get insurance in order and we filled out tons of paperwork. Before we knew it another couple of months had passed us by. We still tried on our own but it seemed futile. We knew there was something wrong with us.

I stared at the calendar counting down the days for our consultation with Dr. Whitworth, our Reproductive Endocrinologist (RE). I continued to chart my cycles. I printed them all (in color of course!), put them in page protectors and put them in my Big Orange Infertility binder. I even gave Eric his own tab that had all of his information. He was mortified. But I felt better. I was prepared. I was ready to take on the next stage of infertility. We were about to start playing with the big dogs.

Big Dogs

I remember the night before our first appointment lying in bed with Eric. One very positive outcome of our infertility journey is that we started praying together each night. We should have been doing it all along but it took this trial to bring us literally to our knees together. I would usually cry and pray for a good 20 minutes. Eric would say a brief heartfelt prayer that was roughly one minute. The night before our appointment, we prayed that God give the doctor wisdom about our situation. We prayed to God to help us have clarity about what to do and what not to do next.

We did not take fertility treatments lightly at all. We certainly were not of the school of thought that fertility treatments were immoral. I believe that God has blessed us with doctors and science that can help make our lives better all around us. If one makes responsible decisions, then that can certainly include fertility treatments. We just wanted to make sure that we were on the path that God wanted us to be on and that we were not just pushing our own baby-making agenda. I was so ready to have a baby and am impatient by nature. I really wanted to make sure that we were doing what God wanted us to do and not just pushing my plan and my timeline.

My first appointment at Nashville Fertility Center was intimidating to say the least. Eric, my big orange binder and I were ushered into an office where we would meet with Dr. Whitworth. We had already filled out a mountain of paperwork about our medical history, etc. before we even got there. Dr. Whitworth wanted to do an ultrasound to determine if she could see what could be causing my irregular cycles.

When she suggested this I thought, "Sure! Let's do this!" Then I walked into the ultrasound room where I was told to undress from the waist down and put a paper blanket across my legs. What?? All the ultrasounds that I had seen on TV were on your belly! Why in the world did I have to take off my pants? AND my undies for that matter! They had to be joking. Insert panic attack *here*. Eric looked every bit as horrified as me. Then when we looked to the side of the table and saw the *wand*, we nearly lost it. Holy Moly. That is going *where??* So I made Eric turn around as I disrobed and covered my shaking legs with the paper blanket. I swear the wait for Dr. Whitworth to come in felt like an eternity. I am sure it was only a couple of minutes, but I was so nervous. Poor Eric looked like he was ready to bolt at any minute. I know he was at war with himself between self-preservation and knowing he had to be a good, supportive husband. If having someone tell you when you can and can't have sex for the last several months hadn't killed the romance, then watching this pelvic ultrasound might be the nail in the coffin.

Dr. Whitworth came in and began to do the ultrasound. I had to be told to scoot down and relax my legs several times. My toes were curled around the stirrups. It was probably the most embarrassing thing I have ever had to do. Little did I know that I would literally have *hundreds* of them over the next several years.

She was able to tell pretty quickly what was causing my abnormal cycles. I had a sizable cyst on my left ovary that had to be removed. This was a cyst that I had had for a while and wasn't caused by the Clomid®. They were able to remove it via an outpatient laparoscopic surgery fairly easily. I remember as I slipped out of consciousness whispering to myself, "One step closer to baby." When I came to after the surgery, I woke to a smiling nurse that said those same words back to me. I thought that was a good sign! I took a long weekend and was able to return to work after that.

Next Steps

Woo hoo! The cyst was gone and we were ready to take our first step in our new fertility plan. Now we just had to wait for a new cycle. Who would know waiting a month would feel like an ETERNITY. Every day looking at the calendar and counting down the days. I felt like I was wishing my life away. One more week. One more day. Was that a cramp? Ugh. Not yet.

Fortunately, I did have a business trip that took me to New York in the midst of the wait. I was close enough to my best friend, Jodi, that I went and spent the weekend with her. She didn't live in the city, but she was close enough that we could drive in. My dad, bless his heart, knew I needed a 'pick me up' and booked us a room so we could stay the night. That gesture meant the world to me. I didn't sit on the

Full Heart Empty Womb

phone and cry to Daddy about not being able to get pregnant, but he still knew my pain. He may not have felt comfortable having a heart to heart with me and quite honestly I wasn't ready to have that conversation with him, either. But he knew that nothing could cheer his baby girl up like the city we both loved with the friend I loved most.

The weekend did so much to help recharge me. It gave me something else to look forward to besides starting my cycle. Spending time with Jodi reminded me about how much I have to be thankful for. Jodi is the most supportive friend in the world. She let me talk and cry when I needed to. Then she pulled my butt into a cab headed to China Town to forget about my worries in search of the perfect handbag. Again, after a glass of wine that night, she held my hand while I got a little teary eyed again.

When I got back I was refreshed and ready to tackle the first step. For me the first step was Intrauterine Insemination - or IUI. Since I responded well to Clomid®, we used that as my follicle stimulating hormone - or FSH. I went in for yet another pelvic ultrasound to determine how many follicles I had and how they were maturing. Everything went just as it was supposed to. We went in for our first IUI feeling very hopeful. Eric was nervous about doing his part. I guess it is the male equivalent of the pelvic ultrasound. He would never talk about it, but I know it was humiliating for him. I admit I had mixed emotions. Sure I felt sorry for him but part of me thought, "Finally he gets a little taste of this!"

The first IUI failed. We were upset of course, but we were ready to try again immediately. We met with Dr. Whitworth and decided we would try three IUIs before we moved on to Invitro Fertilization (IVF).

The doctor also wanted us to do a Sperm Penetration Analysis (SPA). This sounds like a crazy test, but it effectively diagnosed our second major issue with conceiving. Eric provided a sperm sample. They let it sit for 24 hours so that only the strongest, healthiest sperm were left. Then they put them in a dish with *hamster* eggs. This test would simulate an IVF to determine if Eric's sperm could even penetrate an egg. Well we didn't even get to the hamster eggs. After 24 hours all of the sperm had died. So now we have sperm that raced around in circles and didn't even last long enough to find the egg. There really was no hope for us ever conceiving on our own.

We were in the midst of our two-week wait after our second IUI cycle when we got this news. I prayed so hard that it would work and I would get pregnant. We had talked about IVF but really didn't think we would have to go that far. IVF was so much more....everything. More drugs. Needles! Shots! More ultrasounds. More time. More tears. More pressure. More money!

I think the biggest issue for me was that I knew that this was the end of the road, the last step I could take to get pregnant. I really felt deep down in my heart that I would be a mother somehow, some way, some day. But IVF was my last chance to get *pregnant*. To actually have a baby growing in my womb. To have a chance to feel that baby moving and growing inside me. I so desperately wanted to be able to experience that. Was I ready to take that last step? After I took that last step there was no, "But we can still try ...." It was the end of the road of me being able to try to conceive.

After we received another negative result we planned another meeting with Dr. Whitworth. We were just devastated. We had now been pursuing fertility treatments unsuccessfully for almost a year.

Friends were getting pregnant left and right around me. I had shared our struggles with some of my friends. It wasn't necessarily planned. We were at a point in our marriage when people kind of expected you to start a family. Some of my close friends knew we had been trying for a while. They tend to catch on when there are no pregnancy emails coming from you after such a long time! Then it starts to get awkward. They start to tiptoe around you. You either get the announcement where they handle you with kid gloves because they are afraid you are going to explode any minute - or even worse. They don't even tell you. You know that there is a conversation that has taken place; "How do we tell Steph?" How humiliating.

Full Heart Empty Womb

The emotions one struggling with infertility feels when you find out someone else is pregnant are so complex. I was always happy for that person. I would never wish what I was going through on my worst enemy. But did I wish they understood it? Absolutely, but not firsthand. But I was extremely envious. Jealous even. I wanted all of that joy as well instead of the gut wrenching pain that I was enduring. For them this was the happiest time of their life. For me it was the most painful, heartbreaking time. Their pregnancies were turning their Mr. and Mrs. into a family. We were fighting to keep our marriage together and strong so that hopefully someday we could have a family. Then, of course, I would feel guilty for what I felt. Infertility can simply tear you apart emotionally.

The Sunday before our appointment with Dr. Whitworth we decided it was time to confide in some of our closest friends and ask for their prayers. We have a wonderful Sunday school class at our church that is a great support system for us. We asked them to pray for wisdom and peace of mind about our next steps. There were so many directions we could go and I wanted to make sure we took the right path.

We had a great meeting with Dr. Whitworth. We all agreed that in light of the SPA test results, IUIs were not a good option for us. We didn't even know if the sperm could penetrate an egg. The next step for us would be IVF. In addition to IVF we would also do intra-cytoplasmic sperm injection - or ICSI. That is when they actually insert the sperm into the egg. We left the meeting with a great peace about our course of action. I really believe that is a result of the prayers. God didn't audibly say to us, "Stephanie and Eric, thou shalt do IVF!" I believe that the profound sense of peace we felt in a very stressful situation was Him speaking to us. I knew He would not ignore a prayer for wisdom about our decisions.

We decided to take the rest of the year off and enjoy the holidays. The holidays are already a stressful enough time for the infertile even if you aren't doing any treatments! We could start our IVF cycle at the beginning of the New Year. We spent Christmas going between our two families. My sister has two girls and Eric's sister has triplets. Being around the kids at Christmas was hard. Our family was very sensitive to our situation. However I couldn't look at those sweet kids without wondering if we would ever be able to celebrate Christmas with our own kids. I remembered that the year before I just knew I would have a baby by Christmas. Now I was wondering if I ever would. Where will we be next Christmas? Pregnant? Still doing IVF and swimming in medical bills? Would I always just be Aunt Stephie? Would I ever be able to give them the cousins they wanted so badly? And they kept getting older and older! If I ever were able to have kids would they be so old that they wouldn't be close because the age gap had gotten so big? Every night I would cry myself to sleep. I was exhausted. I painted on a happy face all day and held back tears so I wouldn't make anyone uncomfortable or ruin anyone's Christmas. My Mema passed away after Christmas. Now my child would never be able to meet his or her great-grandma. How much more will we miss out on with each passing month?

IVF – Getting Started

January came and we could finally get started with our IVF. Before we started with the actual cycle, our clinic required us both to go to an IVF class that lasted half a day. When we were first told about it I thought, "What in the world are we going to do all that time?" After sitting through it I was so thankful for it. IVF can be very complicated. There are so many different drugs and dosages and the timing is so sensitive. It was great to have a class to really gain understanding of the whole process so that at least that piece of stress was taken off the table. The training on the injections was valuable too. I admit I am a bit squeamish so I tapped Eric on the shoulder and told him that this was his part and took a little mental vacation!

I didn't start my first injections of Lupron until mid-February. My little plan of making Eric be my shot-giving nurse backfired with my first injection. My best friend, Jodi, was having a baby shower out of town on Saturday and that was my first day of Lupron injections. I had given myself permission to miss baby showers for the last several months. It was a survival tactic that served me well. However there was no way I was missing Jodi's shower. She was my best friend and I was happy for her.

I woke up extra early because I knew it would take a little time for me to get the nerve to give myself the shot. It was a subcutaneous shot (Sub Q) where you pinch some skin on your belly and inject yourself right below the skin. That is by no means as difficult or painful as an intramuscular shot (IM) that you give in your hip that goes deep into your muscle tissue. All that being said, if you have a hard time even *looking* at a needle all of that doesn't matter. I called Eric and cried and got a pep talk. I counted to three a gazillion times before I finally took the plunge. Of course I did it way too slow so it hurt more than it should have and I bruised horribly. I called Eric and told him that I did it and we cheered. Pretty ridiculous but it was a big victory for me.

I went to Jodi's baby shower. The whole time I drove there I prayed for strength and the ability to not let my thoughts linger about my infertility during the shower. I just wanted to focus on Jodi. And I didn't want Jodi to feel like she had to focus on me the whole time. The shower was nice. It was primarily her friends from her hometown. She was so sensitive to the fact that it wasn't very easy for me to be there which made me feel guilty too. I hated that because of my infertility she was missing out on some of the joy of her shower. I found her constantly glancing over at me to make sure I was ok. I am so grateful for such a considerate friend. I just hated that even when I was trying my best not to be a wet blanket, I still was because I am infertile.

IVF – Egg Retrieval

The next few weeks went just as we hoped. My body responded well to the drugs and we were hopeful for a positive result. When I had my last ultrasound that showed that my follicles were just about mature, they gave me my HSG shot to take home. Eric had to administer the shot to me that evening at precisely 8:00. The HSG shot would trigger my follicles to release my eggs so they could be retrieved for the IVF. All of my previous shots had been subcutaneous. This would be the first one that would be intramuscular (IM).

Now it had been a couple of months since Eric practiced giving an IM shot and then it was with an orange. I wasn't too excited about him giving it to me. And it was such an important shot that we could not risk it being done incorrectly. Fortunately my nurse friend, Kristen, was ready and willing to help once again! We went over to her house so that she could coach Eric through the shot. After the embryo transfer, I would start to get nightly progesterone injections that would also be IM. It was important for him to feel comfortable administering them. I distinctly remember lying my torso on Kristen's kitchen table with my bottom sticking up in the air. It was nice and numb because I sat on an icepack the whole way to her house. Since she was giving Eric instructions I put my ear buds in so I couldn't hear. At one point I did hear "like a dart" and I promptly turned the Foo Fighters all the way up. To this day I cannot hear "Best of You" without thinking about that moment. It is a fitting song because I feel like I was constantly trying to give the best of me so that I could earn the right just to get pregnant.

I didn't sleep at all the night before the egg retrieval. I was so excited. Since IVF is so expensive we had planned before we even started that this would be our only egg retrieval. We would do only one "fresh IVF" cycle. We would do as many frozen embryo transfers (FET) as we had embryos for. If we hadn't gotten pregnant by then, we would pursue other options. We were not at all opposed to adoption. I just had to at least try and see if we could get pregnant. I wasn't ready to give up that dream. If I couldn't get pregnant, then I would have to mourn that loss before I could take the next step.

Fortunately they were able to retrieve 17 eggs so we were thrilled. We had to wait until noon the next day to see how many, if any, fertilized. The next day we found out that ten of the eggs were mature. They did ICSI on all ten and they fertilized. They also put some of the immature eggs in with the sperm and ONE of them fertilized all on its own with no ICSI! When I called Eric to tell him the results, he was so excited. I think the one sperm that did it all on its own helped his ego tremendously. Sometimes with all of the drama that I had to go through on my own, I would forget about how much this affected him too.

Every day we called to check on the progress of our embryos. Our first goal was to get to three days. Then if they still looked healthy the lab would let them continue to mature before the embryo transfer until day five. I scoured the internet trying to find any promising statistic about what percentage of embryos would make it to day three or day five.

My emotions were across the board during this time. I couldn't believe it. We had embryos! Life! We had never made it this far! I had to believe I was going to get pregnant. How can you put yourself through all of this pain and heartache if you don't truly believe that you can get pregnant? Then of course reality reared its ugly head: it was more likely that the IVF wouldn't work than I would get pregnant this cycle. I teared up and immediately start bawling. Every night I prayed that God would watch over my embryos.

IVF – Embryo Transfer

They gave me a prescription for Valium to take before the procedure to calm my nerves. Eric was just excited that I finally got to pop a pill that made me calm down instead of making me crazy. He was also quite excited about being able to put on scrubs to go into the OR.

The embryologist came to talk to us before the transfer and showed us the picture of our two grade A embryos. They looked like big bubbles with several little bubbles in them but I thought they were precious. I still have that picture in my bedside table. The transfer was a little uncomfortable, but in the grand scheme of things it wasn't too bad.

The worst part of it was post-transfer. I had to go into the transfer with a full bladder so that they could have a clear ultrasound to help with the embryo placement. After being poked and prodded a bit during the transfer, I needed to pee pretty badly. I laid in the bed and stared at the clock willing the 30 minutes to pass more quickly. By the end of the 30 minutes, I was in real pain because I had to go so badly. When I was given the green light to get up, I scurried to the bathroom to relieve myself. I was so scared I was going to pee too hard and lose an embryo! I know it was completely unrealistic, but it was real to me at the time!

I thoroughly enjoyed the bed rest once I got home. Eric rubbed my feet and brought me meals in bed. I couldn't pick up Majors due to the lifting restrictions so we even got him little steps up to the bed. He thoroughly enjoyed me being on bed rest! It wasn't until the next morning that I was over the whole lying around thing. Who knew I would look forward to getting up to pee so much?

I was able to call our voicemail and the embryology lab said they could freeze the four remaining embryos. I was so thankful and *relieved*. This time isn't our only chance! If this IVF didn't work, then we could try one or maybe two FET. When I called Eric to give him the good news, he said exactly what I was thinking. "Everything is going so well for us now, I hope that doesn't mean that it will end soon…" Infertility can make you a pessimist. One is always anticipating failure because most of the time that is all you experience.

Full Heart Empty Womb

I tried to take it easy as best I could during my two week wait between the embryo transfer and my pregnancy test. I didn't want to overdo it physically or take any chances. I worked on my scrapbook from my honeymoon that was three years late. I over analyzed every twinge and cramp I felt. Is that the embryos implanting? Is that an early pregnancy symptom? Or am I about to start my period? My mind was going in overdrive about every little thing.

Eric started doing the progesterone shots in my hip (also known as the upper butt region!). We had a whole routine. I would sit on an ice pack and watch TV while he drew up the meds and got everything ready behind closed doors so I couldn't see any of it. When he was ready I would go in, lean over the vanity, and sing really loudly so I couldn't hear anything. After it was done I would massage in the progesterone because it was so thick and put a heating pad on the area. We would alternate hips so that one side didn't get too sore. I have news for you though. After so many shots, it just hurts everywhere.

My dear friend, Brenda, took me to lunch to help me get my mind off of things one afternoon. We laughed for a solid couple of hours. It was a welcome distraction from all of the stress. She reminded me about a ministry that our church did. I had forgotten that Eric and I had signed up to help that evening. I felt horrible for forgetting our obligation. We had become so self-absorbed with our IVF that we didn't think about much else.

The ministry is called Room in the Inn, and it is a ministry to homeless men. The church picks up ten homeless men from downtown. We feed them supper, let them get showered, pick out new clothes, and sleep in the church's guest house. I went there with every intention of being a blessing to them, but I believe they blessed me tenfold. Those precious men were so gracious and humble.

It was a great reminder of all the many things with which I have been blessed. My road to become a mother wasn't an easy or smooth road. These men had many difficult, bumpy roads in their lives. I had a choice to make. Was I going to be thankful for what I did have? Or was I going to be bitter about what I didn't? I cried the whole way home. I cried because I was thankful for my upbringing and my circumstances that helped me get where I was. I cried of guilt from focusing so much on what I wanted that I didn't have. I had been so self-absorbed the last couple of years. I cried because in spite of it all, I just really wished that I were pregnant. Then I cried even more because my epiphany was so short lived. How cruel the emotions of infertility can be.

The next few days continued to be emotional. Every night I would rest my hands on my belly and talk to my babies. Were they even there? I would pray, bargain with them, whatever I could do to try to make them stick around. "Like that Mexican food? I will make it for you every day!" I would even sing to them as I rubbed my belly. One minute I was up and positive because I was convinced I was pregnant. Then the next minute I was crying hysterically because I was sure I was cramping. I was just emotionally exhausted.

The day before I had the official blood test at the doctor's office I was so tempted to just take a home pregnancy test. The doctors tell you not to take the home pregnancy test because the HSG shot that makes you ovulate can give you a false positive. I felt sure that it was out of my system. I just wanted to KNOW! Eric convinced me to wait. He had planned to take the day off on which I had my pregnancy test at the doctor's office. He wanted to be with me that day whether it was positive or negative. We decided to wait for the official results so we could be there for each other.

Beta Test

As we drove to the fertility clinic the next day, the mood was somber. I told Eric that the next few hours would change the course of our life. Either we would be extremely happy and start planning our future, or we would be even more depressed and continue to wish away our life until the next treatment. I was just so tired of being sad.

They took my blood and I had to wait a few hours for the results. I would call the same voicemail box and get my beta number. Any number over 50 would be considered pregnant. It sounds so personal, huh? Just how I always imagined finding out I was pregnant.

We killed time by going to breakfast. We took the scenic route home, all the while constantly checking the clock. The results would be left on my voicemail box around noon. It was the longest few hours of my life. Finally when it was time we walked to my office to call. I sat on Eric's lap and we said a prayer together through our tears. With shaking hands and blurry eyes I called my voicemail box. "No New Messages." We waited a few minutes and did it again. We called every five minutes until after several attempts we heard, "You have one new message."

We clutched each other tightly and quit breathing while we listened. A cheery voice came on the speaker and said, "Mrs. Greer we are so pleased to tell you that your beta number is 528. You only need 50 to be considered pregnant, so we wonder if you may have two in there! Congratulations. Call to schedule your follow up beta in two days." Click.

Eric and I broke into sobs. I sat on his lap forever, clinging to him as the tears just poured from our eyes. In spite of the impersonal way to finally find out I was pregnant, it was the single most beautiful time in my marriage. I had never seen Eric cry or be overly emotional about anything. In that second I saw all of the pain that he had been shouldering too over the past couple of years. Even though he didn't show it or like to talk about it, he was suffering like I was. And now it was over. I was pregnant!

After we got control of our tears, we called our parents, sisters and the few close friends that knew what was going on. I knew that my mom had been sitting next to the phone for hours waiting for the call. She answered on the first ring with a very tentative, "Hello?" Once we shared the news with her and my dad, I think they cried as hard as we did. It was wonderful. It was almost like the pain of the last couple of years didn't exist for a short while.

We sat down and just enjoyed our good news for a little bit. Then I jumped up and said we had to go. I just couldn't sit around anymore. I was pregnant! I had to go to the one place I had been avoiding the last couple of years – the Target baby aisle! We walked up and down the aisle and giggled and dreamed. We stopped every once and a while and thought, "Is this really real? Or are we just pretending?" Then a cute outfit caught my eye and all was forgotten. Having a baby wasn't a dream anymore. I was actually, finally pregnant!

Chapter Three – A Very Bumpy Road

I wanted to pinch myself. Surely this wasn't real. I went and got my beta tests every other day and watched the numbers grow. It was all good news and I was so thankful. I just stared at the numbers and thought, "This is proof that I am pregnant, right?" It didn't matter that I didn't feel or look any different. Those numbers told me that I was pregnant. Infertility had made me so skeptical that I still had a hard time believing it. When would I feel pregnant? I actually longed for the first morning I would race to the bathroom and throw up from morning sickness.

I didn't realize until I started talking with more ladies going through infertility what a good problem I had. Unfortunately, sometimes ladies can go through fertility treatments and get a positive pregnancy test. However, their beta number isn't as high as they would like it to be or isn't increasing at the rate they expect. Then you are back in the waiting game again. They would have to wait another couple of days to see if their beta numbers increased. You might even have to wait another couple of days to see the result of your third beta test. How heartbreaking. You wait forever to find out yes or no and you get....*maybe*.

First Bump

A couple of weeks after I found out I was pregnant I had a business trip to Cincinnati scheduled for a regional sales meeting. It was the first time I had traveled since my IVF. I couldn't give myself the Intramuscular shots and had needed Eric to administer them to me each night. By this time they had switched the progesterone I was getting nightly from a shot to a suppository. I was excited to get to see some of my dear friends from work. Eric left town as well to go audit a company in Dallas, Texas.

The industry I worked in was very male dominated. There were 23 of us in my sales region, and I was the only female. I was blessed to work with a great group of guys. I only confided in a couple of the guys, Mark and Andy, with whom I had a close friendship, that I was pregnant. They were so excited for Eric and me to have the family we so desperately wanted to have.

One night the entire team went to dinner at a restaurant across from our hotel. During dinner I felt some odd cramps that lasted a few minutes then went away. Immediately it was like all the conversation in the background was 100 miles away. I sat in my seat frozen and thought, "No. No. No. No!!!!!!!!!!!!" It happened again. It took everything in me to not burst into tears and run away. I calmly excused myself and rushed to the ladies room. As soon as I sat down, blood *gushed* from my body. When I looked down I saw a pool of blood and a big clot in the middle. "NO!!!!!!!!!" I stared at the clot and thought, "No God. Please don't let that be my baby!"

I quickly pulled myself together. I sailed by the table and told everyone I was feeling under the weather and rushed back to my hotel room. I felt another cramp and ran straight to the bathroom. Again blood gushed from my body and another clot came out. I panicked and called Eric. I was absolutely hysterical. We couldn't lose our baby after all this! It took a few minutes for him to even be able to understand what I was saying through all the tears and hiccups. He calmed me down and reminded me that my friend, Christy, had experienced bleeding in her pregnancy and that I should call her.

Christy was such a blessing to me. She was also a nurse and she was able to calm me down and get me to think rationally. She had me lie down and take deep breaths. She then encouraged me to call my doctor's after-hours number.

Full Heart Empty Womb

One of the on-call doctors called me back immediately. He was so calm and caring with me and I was so grateful. He had my chart and was able to look at my beta numbers. The doctor told me they couldn't really be sure what happened until I had an ultrasound. He thought that because my beta numbers were so high that if I had indeed had a miscarriage, maybe it was one of the twins. I got an appointment for ten o'clock the next morning for an ultrasound.

That night was the longest of my life. Eric frantically tried to get on the earliest flight back to Nashville. I quickly gathered all my things and drove from Cincinnati to my parents' house in Louisville, Kentucky. I barely remember the two-hour drive. God again watched over me as I drove through my tears. I cried on the phone to Eric and my friend, Kristen. The only prayer I could even get out was, "Please, Lord, please."

When I finally got to my parents' house, my parents were waiting for me. I will never forget the tears and hugs that met me. I looked at their faces and saw broken hearts too. Their hearts broke for their baby and the grandbaby they were so excited to finally have.

My mom laid in bed with me that night and prayed with me. She wrote down a scripture to encourage me. The scripture was Psalm 147:13. "For He strengthens the bars of your gates; He blesses your children within you." I kept that scripture next to me and prayed it continually. That note is still in my Bible today. A calm came over me. I had so many people who were praying for me that night that I know it gave me the peace I needed. I was finally able to pray something more. I prayed, "Lord, please look after my babies. Please put them where it is best for them to be. Whether it is here with us or in Heaven with You. And please help us be at peace with that." If they weren't in my arms, they would be in *His*. My tears slowed down and I fell into a deep sleep.

The next morning my parents drove me the rest of the way to Nashville as I laid down in the passenger seat. My mom and I talked on the way. She said, "Stephanie, you know that God is in control but that doesn't mean that the Devil doesn't intervene to try to hurt you." I pondered that a minute and then said, "Well then the joke is on him because I have prayed more than ever and turned to God during this time!"

Eric got on an early flight. I got to Nashville Fertility Center (NFC) before Eric. I was already back in the ultrasound room before he got there. He came back a few minutes before I had my ultrasound. We clung to each other and cried all the tears that we missed the night before. We gripped each other's hands and prayed with all our might for God's protection over our baby.

Dr. Whitworth came in and did our ultrasound herself. I laid back with tears streaming down the sides of my face as I gripped Eric's hand. I prayed Psalm 147:13 in my head over and over as she moved the wand to try to find a baby.

And then she did. She found a baby *with a heartbeat!* Then she found another baby *with a heartbeat!* And then she found a sub chorionic hemorrhage (SCH) that was right next to my cervix. It was also right next to one of the babies and was twice the size of it!

I dressed and we met with Dr. Whitworth to discuss the ultrasound. We were so excited. We had not only one, but two babies with heartbeats! They were alive!! However, we were anxious to hear about the SCH. It looked like a huge blob that was ready to gobble up my babies and I was scared.

Dr. Whitworth told me that I had to take it easy and let it heal. It could take a couple of weeks or months. With time, hopefully the clot would heal and be absorbed into my uterus. I would go home on bed rest and come back the following week for another ultrasound. She also switched me back to taking progesterone via an IM shot until the end of my first trimester.

Another long week of bed rest and lots of prayers. I took my doctor's orders very seriously. I stayed in bed except to shower, potty, and throw up. Yes, my morning sickness finally reared its ugly head! I still cramped and spotted some, but it gradually lessened.

When I went back for my follow up ultrasound, we saw that the babies had grown to twice their size! The SCH was still there, but it was getting smaller. It was still way too close to Twin A. I went home and did the same thing again, hopeful for better news the next week. By the end of two weeks the SCH had been completely absorbed by my uterus!

We were so grateful. Finally I felt like I could *enjoy* being pregnant. I also let myself really think about and revel in the fact that we were going to have *twi*ns! I had been hesitant to think about it too much before because I was so scared that we were going to lose one of them. People ask me all the time what I thought when I found out that we were having twins. I felt nothing but absolute, pure joy.

The next few months were rather boring and quite wonderful! I registered for all those precious things that I either avoided or cried about while I struggled to get pregnant. I thoroughly enjoyed the whole concept of eating for *three*. Eric and I went on a little baby moon to the beach. We just reveled in being in our happy place.

Since I was pregnant with twins, I went to a high-risk obstetrician for regular ultrasounds. We were thrilled when we learned that Twin A was a boy and Twin B was a girl. One of each! How perfect! The best news though was that they looked perfectly healthy.

Big Bump...and not just my Belly

One day I went in for my regular ultrasound and checkup. I had been through so many at this point that I was borderline relaxed. I would throw my arm behind my head and make myself comfortable. I had pretty much mastered the art of awkward conversation with my feet up in stirrups and an ultrasound tech chatting away in between my legs. The conversation would vary between the hot summer and if I was nervous about having twins. This day we chatted over Eric's and my anniversary plans for that night.

Full Heart Empty Womb

The conversation stopped somewhat abruptly. She looked a little concerned and asked if I was having contractions. I quickly shook my head no. She told me to get dressed and quickly left the room. I got dressed, confused about what just happened. I had not felt any different at all. I was only 22 weeks. There was no way I was having any contractions. What in the world could she have seen? It didn't take long for my panic to take hold and I started to tear up.

The ultrasound tech came back in and told me to go immediately to my OB, Dr. Blake's, office. I called Eric in a panic on the way over to her office. Once I got there the receptionist ushered me straight back to Dr. Blake's personal office. She told me to lie down on the couch. I was officially in full-blown panic and the tears were flowing freely now.

Dr. Blake came into the office and sat with me on the couch. She held my hand and explained to me that my cervix had shortened dramatically in the last couple of weeks. One of the causes for a shortened cervix was contractions. I was stunned. There was no way I was having contractions. Again, I was only 22 weeks. Granted I was measuring a little bigger than that since I was carrying twins but not that much. I couldn't be having contractions yet! I didn't feel a single thing.

She had me admitted for monitoring at the Women's Hospital next door. I made yet another panicked call to Eric to come and meet me at the hospital. I called my parents, my sister, and all my prayer warriors to jump into action.

They hooked me up to monitors, tested my urine, and took blood. It didn't take long to see on the monitor that I was having contractions. And not just one here and there. I was having contractions every seven minutes. And the scary part was I never felt a single one.

Eric sat next to me and held my hand. We were so thankful that I was having regular ultrasounds so that they caught the contractions. How long would I have had them before I noticed?

Full Heart Empty Womb

If I had gone into labor at 22 weeks the babies would not have even been *viable*. *Viable*. That is a scary word. I had never heard it in relation to a baby before that day. Viable means that the baby has reached a stage in development where the fetus has even a remote chance of survival outside of the uterus. Most doctors would not even intervene before a baby is viable. A baby is not considered viable until 24 weeks gestation.

The nurses and doctors sprang into action to get my contractions under control. I was admitted overnight for observation. I was under strict orders to lie flat and on my left side. I wasn't supposed to get up except to go to the restroom. I was also told that I had to drink a lot of water to make sure I was not dehydrated.

They gave me a drug, Terbutaline®, through my IV to help stop the contractions. The drug made my whole body shake and my heart race. I was miserable. I had never felt quite like this. It was like I wanted to get up and run laps to get out some of the shakes but I couldn't. I just had to lie there and drink water.

And drinking water while I was lying flat? Not an easy feat. My hands were shaking and I would lift my head a little to take a big gulp through the straw. Half of it would end up on my pillow. The nurses kept coming in to refill my big pink jug of water and encouraged me to drink more and more.

Then they would come in over the intercom on my bed (yes, and I jumped the first time that happened!) and say, "Mrs. Greer you need to go empty your bladder. A full bladder can cause contractions." I couldn't win. Eric would help me out of bed and unplug my IV pole. I would quickly go to the restroom and hurry back to lie down and chug more water.

Over time though, all of this effort seemed to help slow the contractions. Since it was our anniversary, Eric went to get us some carry out to enjoy in our room. He laid in bed with me as we prayed for our babies. We were scared, but we knew we were in the right place.

All night I continued with the same routine. Drink. Pee. Drink. Drink. Pee. Get a bolus shot of the medicine. Shake. Sweat. Drink. Spill my water. Drink. Pee. I didn't sleep a wink that night.

At one point the backup battery died on my IV pole. Every time we unplugged it for me to go to the restroom, it beeped at me. We laughed that we thought it sounded like the beeps in between commercials on our favorite TV show, *24*. As if I needed any more pressure! Lie down flat! But not on your back because that can cause contractions. Don't get up! Being up can cause contractions. Drink so you don't get dehydrated! But don't let your bladder get full because that will cause contractions. So I get up to go to the bathroom. Beep…..beep….beep!!! Get back in bed. And around and around it went all night.

By morning the contractions had slowed down but hadn't gone away completely. They were comfortable enough to release me. I went home on bed rest with strict orders. I was only able to get up to go to the bathroom and to shower once a day. I also was given an oral form of the medicine that I had been given via IV. I was to go back for another ultrasound the following week to check my progress. I learned that if the contractions slowed then my cervix could actually lengthen. I was determined to follow the directions perfectly so that my cervix would get longer by next week.

It was a long week at home. It was hard for me because I never felt any of the contractions. Was I having them? Was I doing everything right? I certainly felt the negative side effects of the drugs, but were they doing what they were supposed to do and slowing down the contractions?

I stayed in bed and never got up except when I was allowed. Eric packed snacks next to my bed so I didn't have to get up. I refilled my water when I got up to go to the restroom. My brother-in-law, Jamie, came by to check on me and bring me lunch in bed. I even skipped my beloved shower one day because I was afraid I had been up too many times to go to the restroom.

When I went back for my follow up ultrasound I was hopeful that my cervix had lengthened. I was a model patient. I had done everything that was asked of me. Besides that Eric and I prayed incessantly over our babies. I spent hours crying, rubbing my belly, and begging God to please keep them safe in my belly for weeks to come.

I was so nervous by the time I had my ultrasound. I had been up out of bed for an hour between showering, traveling to the doctor's office, and waiting for my ultrasound. That was the longest I had been out of bed in over a week.

Unfortunately the ultrasound showed that my cervix had gotten even shorter in the last week. We drove over to Dr. Blake's office and I cried and cried. As soon as we walked into the office they again ushered me straight back to her personal office for me to lie on her couch. Eric held my hand and reassured me that everything would be ok.

Dr. Blake came in and took my other hand and told me that she was admitting me to the hospital. I likely wouldn't go home until after I delivered the babies. Her nurse came in with a wheelchair to take me straight to the hospital.

Permanent Resident

I cried on the way over to the hospital. It was too soon. We still weren't to the point of viability yet. Then an overwhelming sense of peace washed over me. I was never able to feel the contractions. If I was in the hospital, I knew they could monitor me and try to keep them under control.

My friend, Kristen, came to my aid again. She was a labor and delivery nurse, but she also worked on the high-risk pregnancy floor. She was familiar with their protocols. She assured me that they had many different ways that they could intervene to help keep my contractions under control so we could make it to viability. I clung to that. I didn't let myself believe that those words were anything but complete and total FACT.

The second day we were there we met with a nurse from the Neonatal Intensive Care Unit (NICU). That was overwhelming. I had just gotten to a place of peace that we would get our babies to the point of viability. A point where they would just have a chance to *live*. She spoke in very vague terms about the numerous complications we could face if the babies were born in the next couple of weeks.

We toured the NICU and I saw babies that were absolutely tiny in incubators. They had tubes and IVs coming out from every direction. I teared up and asked how far along they were. 27 weeks. 28 weeks. They were all *months* older than my babies were now. I finally understood why she was being so vague. My babies were still a long, long way away from even being one of her smallest babies in the NICU. I felt utterly defeated.

Dr. Blake came to visit me in the hospital every morning. She noticed my somber mood and gave me a pep talk. We got a calendar and put it up on my bulletin board in my room. We set a goal to get to 24 weeks. Every morning I got a big red marker and crossed off a day. Once we got to 24, we would reach for 26. After 26, we would shoot for 28 and so on. She encouraged me that every day I kept my babies in my belly was four less days that they would be in the NICU. I was a better incubator than any incubator they had in that state of the art NICU downstairs.

Now that was some real motivation. I was going to fight. I had to fight to get pregnant. Now I was going to fight to stay pregnant. I was going to fight every single day so that my babies would then get their chance to fight.

Full Heart Empty Womb

There was no time for me to sit around and feel sorry for myself. I had to stay strong. This is what I cried and prayed for so many nights. I wanted to be pregnant. Sure I never imagined that my pregnancy would be riddled with so much pain, but it didn't matter. I was pregnant with my babies. Now it was time for me to be strong for them and focus on what I could do.

The days were long. I had to lie with my bed flat. The only time I could have any incline was when I ate my meals. I alternated between lying on my sides. I couldn't lie on my back because that would cause even more contractions. Sometimes I would accidentally roll onto my back in my sleep. I would be awakened by a nurse coming over my intercom saying, "Mrs. Greer, you are contracting more. Are you lying on your side? Or do you need to go empty your bladder?"

I was on the same medications to slow my contractions but on a higher dose. My hands shook and my heart raced. I couldn't read because it was hard for my eyes to focus on the words let alone even hold a book. I tried to work on the Christmas stockings I was going to make for the babies. My hands shook so much that I couldn't even hold the materials without dropping them. I had sequins all over me and my bed. So as a result, I watched a lot of TV. My high point of the day was when I got to eat lunch and watch The Young and the Restless.

My body felt like it was on fire most of the time. I had my air turned as low as it would go. I would wear my tank top and shorts and watch people bundle up as they came in my room. I hated that they were uncomfortable but I loved the company. My mother-in-law, Sarah, and sister-in-law, Amy, were so good about coming to sit with me.

Sarah and Amy were familiar with this whole routine. It had only been a few years before that Amy was in a similar situation when she was pregnant with triplets. Amy was admitted to the hospital at 27 weeks and stayed on bed rest until she delivered Houston, Madeline and Elizabeth at 31 weeks and 5 days. They were intimately aware of the struggles I was going through.

I am so thankful for the wonderful family I married into. They would take turns coming and sitting with me to keep me company during the day. They would always bring me lunch and lots of conversation to keep my mind off of things. My father-in-law, Brent, would come by to see me any time he had a meeting in Nashville. They understood how lonely being in the hospital long term could be.

The longest hours of the day were from 4:00 pm to about 6:30 pm when Eric would get to the hospital. By then I was beyond tired of lying in a bed and it was too early to go to sleep. There was never anything I was too interested in watching on TV. I would be so desperate some days that I actually watched "Everybody Loves Raymond" in Spanish. I spent hours either staring at the contraction monitor or the horrible vine wallpaper border in my room. On one wall the pattern repeat didn't match, and it about drove me out of my little OCD mind! I dreamed about climbing up there and ripping it down.

Day by day we marked off the days on the calendar. My cervix seemed to be steady. It wasn't getting any longer, but it wasn't getting much shorter. It seemed that we had found the right mix of medication and bed rest that had at least slowed the contractions.

Viability Vacation

On the day I got to 24 weeks, I felt the weight of the world lift from my shoulders. I knew we still had a very long road ahead of us, but we had made it to our first goal. Since I had been fairly steady, they actually started talking about releasing me and letting me continue my bed rest at home.

As much as this excited me, I was still a little nervous at the prospect of going home. When I was at the hospital I had the comfort of the monitors. Granted being hooked up to monitors was anything but comfortable, yet they were very reassuring. I had learned how to read the contraction monitoring tape. I could look and see how many I was having and how far apart they were. Since I still couldn't feel my contractions, it was very reassuring to me.

That being said, when I made it to 26 weeks and they released me, I would have jumped up and clicked my heels if it were allowed. I was released to go home on the same drugs on bed rest for at least a little while. The doctors prepared me that I would most likely have to come back. I would go back for an ultrasound in a week. They would measure my cervix to see if it shortened and indicated more contractions. I was grateful for whatever time I had at home.

On the drive home Eric put the passenger seat all the way down. We had to stop at a gas station to get me a bottle of water because Heaven forbid I drive 20 minutes home without drinking any water. I distinctly remember being at the gas station parked next to a very stinky dumpster. That didn't matter to me though. I was so happy to finally breathe in some fresh air. I had happy tears streaming down my face as I praised God for watching over me and my babies.

The doctors set me up with home health care so that I could do some monitoring at home. I had to monitor my pulse to make sure that my heart rate wasn't getting too high. For some reason that was very hard and stressful for me. I never could get my pulse right. I also had to monitor my blood pressure. I had a very interesting contraction monitor that I would wear a couple of times a day. After I wore it I would plug it into a telephone line, and my results would be faxed to a nurse to read.

The best part of being home was that Eric and I got to lie in bed together each night. Eric was the most supportive husband ever. There was only one night that he didn't spend with me, sleeping on the vinyl pull out couch in the hospital. On that night I had to practically push him out. I begged him to take some laundry home so I could have some clean clothes. Really I just wanted him to have a decent night's sleep. The clean undies were a bonus.

At home we got to lie in bed and snuggle. He got to lie next to me with his hands on my belly and talk to the babies. We laid together and prayed for the babies as we felt them move beneath our hands. Sure, we did that at the hospital, but there was something more intimate about it when he wasn't sitting in a hospital chair next to my bed. I cried every night because I was so thankful to be home if even for just a little while.

On the morning of my ultrasound I packed my bag ready to go back to the hospital. I was hopeful that I would go back home, but I had realistic expectations. Honestly, although I loved being at home, it was also stressful for me. Since I never felt any of my contractions, I often worried that I was contracting more and didn't even know it. The home health care was great, but it wasn't as reliable as being in the hospital. If they saw that I was contracting more in the hospital, they could react immediately.

One-Way Ticket

I was not surprised at all when I went to my ultrasound and saw that my cervix had shortened. They could even see a contraction during the ultrasound. I had gotten a one-way ticket back to the high-risk maternity floor. The next time I would leave the hospital would be after I delivered the babies.

Eric wheeled me up to the seventh floor in my wheel chair. I went to the nurses' station and saw the sweet, familiar faces that I had come to know so well over the last month. I could see the mix of disappointment and happiness to see me again. They were sad that I had to come back, but we had formed a nice friendship while I was there.

Since we were hoping for a nice long stay on the floor, the nurses arranged for me to be put in the big room at the end of the hallway. My real estate would be the same no matter what - a hospital bed - but

Full Heart Empty Womb

Eric would be much more comfortable. We joked that my hospital room was our apartment in the city. We lived way out in the suburbs of Nashville and Eric usually had at least a 30-minute commute. The company he was auditing was just down the street from the hospital so it was actually pretty convenient for him! It was also nice for me to have him so close just in case I needed him.

The coming days and weeks were more of the same. I lived from ultrasound to ultrasound. I held my breath to see how long my cervix was. They measured my amniotic fluid to make sure it didn't get too low because one of the medications I was on could lower it. They looked at several factors to see if they needed to alter my medication and to see how I was progressing.

My favorite part was when I got to actually see the babies. Often times they had to tell me what I was looking at but it didn't matter. I could stare at them all day. Every other week they would measure the babies to try to figure out their weights. It took a while for them to find and measure the various bones that they would use to calculate their weight. I had to be lying on my back and it was extremely uncomfortable. By the end of it the ultrasound tech was always apologizing and I was holding back tears.

I would wait each morning to see the doctors and hear their thoughts. I would pepper them with questions. How long do you think I will make it? How much shorter can my cervix get? What is the next step with my meds? They generally gave me very vague answers. I understand it was because we were dealing with a very fluid situation and things could change on a dime, but it was frustrating. Then I would call my family to give them an update and get peppered with the same questions. It was exhausting.

We did what we could to make the most out of a bad situation. It was football season so Saturday was no longer a boring day on TV for me. My sister-in-law, Amy, even made me some chili and rotel to eat one night as we watched the UT football game. My friends planned a baby shower. They arranged for me to get a wheelchair pass for an hour.

Full Heart Empty Womb

They set up the shower in the family lounge for us all to gather in. For one hour I felt normal. I opened gifts with sweet little outfits and other baby things. I finally was able to let myself smile and think about having healthy babies. The next day my Sunday school class had a shower for me too. Although the doctors would have allowed it, I was too scared to be up any more that weekend. We crammed 20 women in my room so I could stay lying down and celebrated my babies some more. I was so grateful for a little bit of normalcy.

Since we were getting ready to have twins, we decided that it was time to trade in my sedan and get a minivan. We had kind of looked around early on in my pregnancy, so I knew that a minivan was what I wanted. I could fit two babies in my back seat no problem. It was all the gear that went with them that was the problem! The double stroller took up my entire trunk. Heaven forbid I wanted to put anything else in there because there was no room at all.

We looked online at various used minivans. Thank God there are so many websites that have so many pictures. I actually felt like I was a part of picking out my new wheels. The gentleman that was going to sell us the minivan also wanted to buy my car. Dr. Blake was kind enough to write orders for me to be able to take a wheel chair ride down to the parking lot to say goodbye to my beloved car.

I was excited to be getting my minivan. A minivan symbolized being a Mom to me and that was all I ever wanted. However, I worked my tail off to earn the money to buy my first car. I loved it. So there I was sitting in my wheelchair, crying next to another stinky dumpster, patting the trunk of my beloved car. A week later I got another Get Out of Jail pass to take a ride to the parking lot again. This time it was all happy tears for my silver Minivan. I would take my babies home in this vehicle!

Home Stretch

Each day I got up, crossed my day off, and thanked God for watching over us one more day. When I got to week 30, I finally started to breathe a little easier. By then the babies had a very good chance of not only surviving but not having any significant developmental issues.

I was very fortunate to live in Nashville. I didn't realize this fact but Nashville is actually quite the medical community mecca. I was blessed to be under the care of an entire team of high-risk obstetricians. In addition to Dr. Blake, the other OBs also came to see me every day. Their main goal was to keep me pregnant another day so that my babies would have a chance to develop as much as possible before delivery.

They have had thousands of patients and held a wealth of knowledge. As a result, I was on a specific drug regimen that was tailored to my specific issues. I was on several different drugs, but the main one remained to be Terbutaline® from the time I went into the hospital. Instead of being on an IV, they put me on a continual low dose via an infusion pump. I still had a bolus dose every few hours. The device was similar to what a diabetic would wear. Mine was through my thigh. The side effects never really got better. I just learned to live with them. I had spots all over my leg from the various infusion sites.

Around 31 weeks my contractions were getting worse and worse. My cervix was nearly non-existent. The high-risk doctors decided it was time to go for the final straw – Magnesium Sulfate. Otherwise known as "Mag." Most hospitals will only put a patient on Mag for a few hours or administer a bolus shot. I would be put on an IV for a considerably longer time.

The side effects of Mag are dramatic. I believe that is why most patients are only on the drug for a short amount of time. The side effects were similar to Terbutaline® but amplified 100 times. Literally. My body felt like it was on FIRE. If I didn't have people coming in and out of my room, I would have just completely stripped. Instead I lived in a tank top and shorts. I took cold showers and left my hair wet to help me cool down. Eric even bought me a couple of fans. We turned them on high and had them blowing directly on me at all times. I also had the shakes pretty bad. I do think that being on Terbutaline® for so long helped me get used to the shaking. It was manageable.

The entire time I was in the hospital I was positive and upbeat. I never complained. I was ready to stand on my head if they told me to. This is what I wanted. I was their mama. I had to do whatever I had to do to protect them. Now my job was to lie in a hospital bed no matter how miserable I was.

All that being said, I was finally to the point where I felt *broken*. I had been in the hospital on bed rest for two months. Before I got pregnant I was a petite girl who weighed 110 pounds. I gained over 60 pounds. I don't say that out of vanity. I say that to point out it is a lot of weight on a small frame! I was beyond uncomfortable. I hurt all over and there was *nothing* that I could do about it. There were two positions in which I could lie and after 5 minutes I got uncomfortable.

One day the lady that cleaned my room came in to mop. I had been crying a little bit and was embarrassed. There was no such thing as privacy when you lived in a hospital. I quickly wiped my tears so that she wouldn't feel uncomfortable. I painted on my happy face ready to shoot the breeze as she mopped away.

I leaned over to grab my water off the table. She said, "Shoowee Girl! I didn't realize you had those!!". I asked her what she was talking about and she said, "All those stretch marks on your hips!" At that point I wasn't concerned with making her uncomfortable. I just let the tears roll.

As soon as she left the room I called Eric bawling. The poor thing had jumped every time he saw my number come up on his caller id for months. He would answer the phone in a panic. "Hey are you ok? Are you ok?" I cried and told him about my hurt feelings. He sighed in relief and like a good husband told me how beautiful and strong I was.

I dealt with extreme guilt. I was encouraged every day by the nurses and doctors. "Every day you keep your babies in your belly is four less days in the NICU!" I knew that. I clung to that. But a growing part of me was just *done*. And that made me feel completely horrible. After all, I had to stay strong for my babies.

One day Eric came home - to the hospital - with a present for me. Inside was a necklace and a pair of earrings with opals. October's birthstone. It was already the second week in October. I was so touched by his thoughtfulness. I knew he was desperately trying to cheer me up. There was something else in that gift though. I felt like in his own way he was telling me it was ok. It was ok if I only lasted a couple more weeks. It was ok if the babies were born in October. In fact he expected it. I had fought a good fight. That gift gave me the strength to hold on a little while longer.

Shortly after that time, they saw that my contractions were continuing to get worse. They increased my Mag dosage to what I thought was the maximum. The side effects continued to get worse. Every day felt like an eternity. I would lie in bed with one hand on my belly and the other fingering the opal necklace on my chest praying day in and day out.

One Sunday afternoon my in-laws came to visit us on their way through Nashville. It was so good to see them. However my back really started to hurt while they were there. Eric had gotten me a heating pad and I had it strapped onto my back trying to get relief from the pain. By that night I felt sick to my stomach and had no appetite. The pain started to stretch from my back through my belly so that I just hurt everywhere. I had to get up several times because I felt like I was going to throw up or pee. I didn't sleep a wink that night and neither did Eric.

October 16 – The Day That Should Have Been

When the morning nurse came in, she could tell immediately that I was in a lot of pain. The normal positive Stephanie was gone. I just cried and told her I was done. I couldn't do it anymore. Those were the hardest words for me to ever say. I felt like I was giving up. I just couldn't do it anymore. I was in so much pain. She assured me that it was her goal that day to get me to deliver my babies. She told me to not eat anything. I was having a C-section and it would have been delayed if I had eaten within a certain timeframe. I didn't have an appetite anyway.

I was so relieved. I called my mom and told her that I thought today was finally going to be the day. Eric called his parents and the telephone tree sprang into action. We waited anxiously for the doctors. I didn't even get up for my daily shower because I just knew as soon as I got in the shower the doctor would walk in and I would miss my chance to talk to him.

The doctor and nurse came in a couple of hours later. Eric had been pacing the floors and I was tossing in bed trying to get comfortable. We both sprang to attention when they walked through the doors. He looked at my file and made a couple of notes. Then he turned to my nurse, my would-be savior, and told her to up my Mag dosage again. What??? I thought I was already on the highest dosage!

I cried to him and repeated that I couldn't do it anymore. I pleaded with him. I was 32 weeks and 4 days. I had been in the hospital on bed rest on massive amounts of drugs for 10 weeks and 4 days and never complained. I took every order they had given with a smile. Today I was done.

He gave me the same speech about every day equaling four fewer days in the NICU. I felt smaller than a flea. I decided to change tactics then. I begged for something to help with the nausea. I wanted something to help me get some much needed sleep. He granted me that request and marched on to the next room.

I felt so defeated. In a flash I went from so excited to finally get to meet my babies to facing who knew how much longer of pain. I had Eric make the calls to let everyone know it was a false alarm. I couldn't talk.

The nurse came in with the same defeated look on her face. She apologized and rubbed my arm as she changed the setting on my IV of Mag. She administered some Phenergan to help with the nausea and gave me something to help me sleep.

I was finally able to sleep but only for about 20 minutes at a time. I would shoot up and feel like I was about to throw up. I would get out of bed and rush as much as I could to the bathroom. It is not easy to rush when you are drugged up, as big as a house, and attached to an IV pole and fetal monitor. After a while I was so woozy that I could barely even walk, so Eric had to practically carry me each time to the bathroom. This routine lasted all day and all night.

October 17 – Welcome to the World

The next morning they had me attached to the fetal monitors for a while. I was borderline delirious because I hadn't had any real sleep in almost 48 hours. I was also still in an enormous amount of pain. Lying on my side for the monitoring was excruciating. They were starting to talk about delivering again because the babies were not responsive. They still had a strong heartbeat but they were lethargic....much like their mommy.

Dr. Blake came in to visit me. She was immediately alarmed when she looked at me. I told her about the pain. She asked me if I minded if she checked me for dilation. When she checked me, I was four

Full Heart Empty Womb

centimeters dilated. It was finally time to have my babies. My tears of pain and agony turned to tears of relief and happiness.

We sprang into action again. The phone tree was activated. My dad had just gotten on a plane to Chicago, so he boarded a plane home as soon as he landed. My sister, Amy, made plane reservations to fly down later that week. Everyone else hopped in the car to Nashville.

Within no time at all the anesthesiologist came to administer my spinal tap. I remember he kept trying to get me to hunch over a little more so he could get it in the right spot. I am pretty sure I had a smart aleck reply about not being able to hunch over much more with my huge belly!

I laid back in bed and waited for them to whisk me away to the operating room. Eric still paced the room with a crazy look in his eyes. He had been through the emotional and physical ringer the last couple of days too. He didn't get much more sleep than I. I also cannot imagine how difficult it would be to watch someone you love go through so much pain and not be able to do anything about it.

I was wheeled into the operating room with happy tears running down the sides of my face. I had made it. Praise the Lord for giving me the strength to get through the last eleven weeks.

There was a crowd of about 20 people in there. There was Dr. Blake and her nurses. The NICU staff was there with an incubator ready to transport the babies to the NICU after delivery. I had also consented to have some nursing students come in to observe the delivery. I guess I was a good learning case for them!

At 11:07am Ethan Brent Greer was born weighing a hefty four pounds four ounces. One minute later Ella Bailey Greer was born weighing four pounds. I didn't get to hold or kiss either of them. I got a quick look at them in the incubator. They each had a nurse who had them bagged and was helping them breathe. And just like that they were gone to the NICU.

Final Thoughts

People may hear about my difficulty getting pregnant with Ethan and Ella and think I was pushing fate when we decided to go through fertility treatments. Maybe God just didn't want us to have babies. After hearing about my struggles to just stay *pregnant*, they may think that we were still pushing something that just wasn't meant to be. Maybe we just weren't meant to be parents. It was a very bumpy road getting to here. Aren't most of the roads worth traveling anything but smooth?

Today Ethan and Ella are healthy, normal eight year olds. They just started second grade. They have already been a blessing to our lives and to so many others' lives. I can look at them today and see the potential that they have. Ethan is a little math genius like his Daddy and that makes me so proud. But it is his caring heart that brings me to my knees. Every night he prays from his heart for several people. I listen to his heartfelt prayers and know that he is straight from God. He tells me he wants to be a doctor or go into the military. How many lives will my baby save because we were brave enough to fight for his?

Ella has a love for reading like her Mama. She is always asking for five more minutes with her book before bed. But it is her nurturing heart that brings tears to my eyes. Since she has been in preschool, she has always had at least one special needs child in her class. Ella always gravitates to them. She never looks at them as different. She just wants to be their friend and help them. She tells me that she wants to be a teacher when she grows up. I can see her being a special education teacher like her Aunt Sharon. How many lives will she touch because we didn't give up on hers? I also know without a doubt that she will be a wonderful mother. How many more generations of children will come from us because we didn't give up on our family?

God was at work in our very bumpy road. He never guaranteed us or anyone a smooth road to parenthood or anything else for that matter.

This bumpy road taught me so many lessons that make me a better mom, wife, and daughter in Christ that I would never take for granted...

Chapter Four – Highs & Lows

After they took Ethan and Ella to the NICU, I smiled at Eric and said, "We did it" then immediately passed out. I was in and out of consciousness the rest of the day. I would wake up for a minute and mutter something incoherent and then pass out again. Every time I woke up there was someone else sitting in my room. They were on "Steph Watch". At one point I passed out in the middle of a sentence while talking to my mom and woke up finishing the sentence to my brother-in-law, Jamie. It was a bizarre day but it was a blessing. I was so out of it that I wasn't aware that I couldn't go see my babies in the NICU. Everyone in my family had seen them but me.

Late in the day a lactation consultant came in to help me start pumping. I could hardly stay awake, but by gosh I was going to start pumping my babies some milk. It was the least I could do to help them grow big and strong. The consultants set me up on a three-hour rotation around the clock to help me build up my milk supply. We set the alarm to wake us up. Eric would set up the pump for me and go check on the babies while I pumped. We passed out and did it all over again about two and a half hours later. Barely anything came out when I pumped, but I was assured that it was "liquid gold" and was essential for my sweet babies.

I woke up the next morning finally feeling a little more human. I could move my legs and actually stand up. I had to wait to see the doctor before I could go downstairs to the NICU. I made the most of my time by eating a breakfast like I hadn't eaten in three days and taking a glorious shower.

As soon as I got the all clear, I put on my robe ready to WALK to the NICU to finally get to meet my sweet babies. It was just down the hall to the elevator but it was the farthest I had walked in almost three months. By the time I got down there I felt like I needed a nap.

Eric showed me how to wash all the way up to my elbows and helped me put on all the protective clothing required to go into the NICU. It was pretty intimidating. Ethan and Ella's beds were all the way in the back of the NICU. We walked softly through the room. It was fairly quiet except for the constant beeps of the various monitors attached to all of the babies.

Love at First Sight

We finally made it back to their beds. Happy tears streamed down my face. My babies. Oh, my sweet babies. They were so tiny and perfect. Their preemie diapers were so big on them that they were nearly folded in half and still went halfway up their chests. Their little legs didn't have a single roll on them. Their cheeks had no chubbiness. Their little preemie-sized pacifiers still took up half of their faces. And they were just perfect.

My mom was with Ella so I gave her a quick kiss on the head and walked to stand with Ethan. The NICU had a limitation of one or two visitors per bed to avoid crowding and to keep the noise level down for the babies.

I walked over to meet my son, Ethan. "Hi Buddy. It's Mommy." I choked out the word. *Mommy*. "I've been missing you." He turned his little head and locked his beautiful brown eyes with mine. For the second time in my life, I fell in love with someone as soon as our eyes met.

I wanted so badly just to scoop him up. I wanted just to love on him and shower him with a million kisses. But I couldn't. In fact I had to be very careful about even touching him. A preemie could be easily startled. I warmed up my hands and slowly put my hand next to his. His tiny fingers gripped my finger. Yes. This. This is what the last two years were all about. This makes every tear, prayer, shot, and day in bed worth it. My *baby*.

Full Heart Empty Womb

My mom came to switch places with me so I could meet my sweet girl. Ella was awake, too. She turned when she heard me whisper to her. "Oh, my sweet girl. How I love you so. Mommy is here." Her beautiful blue eyes blinked, slowing taking me in. I wanted to rain little kisses all over her sweet face and little belly. Instead I warmed up my hand and carefully put one on the top of her head and one on her little frog legs. The NICU nurses said that this made them feel safe like in a little cocoon. I could stare at my sweet girl for days.

Eric came in to trade places with Mimi. Yes, my mom had made the transition to Mimi now! Since Eric and I were both there the nurses let us help with their bottles. As much as I wanted to be able to nurse, they were just not strong enough. Because they were so small, we couldn't risk them exerting too much effort and burning more calories than they were taking in.

The nurse handed me the tiniest bottle I have ever seen. It looked like a bottle that I had for one of my dolls when I was little. The tiny bottle was only filled up about halfway. We could only attempt to feed them by the bottle for a few minutes. Since they were premature, they had not had the opportunity to really develop the suck and swallow reflex that is learned in utero. They got tired pretty quickly and fell asleep as they were trying to drink their bottles. We put the rest in their feeding tubes so they wouldn't exert too much energy.

They were already getting stronger. Their first day they were on a ventilator, but by this time they were already moved to just a nasal cannula. I, on the other hand, still had a long way to go. My little excursion to the NICU had left me wiped out. Eric could tell I was in pain and suggested I go back up to my room to rest. I protested and he assured me we could come right back down after I rested. I kissed my babies, and he helped me hobble back upstairs.

By the time I made it back to my room, I was ready to pass out. Between recovering from the C-section and bed rest I was incredibly weak. I was pumping every three hours around the clock, so Eric helped get my pump set up before I laid down for a little bit. I wasn't tired because I slept most of the day before. It took a lot of effort for me to force myself to lie down for a while. I wanted to be downstairs with my babies. The nurses strongly encouraged me to lie down for at least a couple of hours so I wouldn't overdo it.

That tended to be our routine over the next few days. I would pump in my room. I would rest a little bit and give the nurses a chance to check me out. As soon as I could, I would go down to the NICU to sit with my babies. If I had any time in between I would walk up and down the halls to try to regain my strength.

When Ethan and Ella were a couple of days old, they both got jaundiced. The nurses put them under a bilirubin light and put the little glasses on them. We were already really restrictive about how much we could hold them, and this condition hampered it even more. I would just sit next to their beds and gaze at how cute they looked in their little glasses.

When their jaundice improved, we got to start a new therapy with them called, "Kangaroo Care". During Kangaroo Care we would hold the babies in nothing but their diapers. We would hold them inside our shirts, skin to skin. This position helped them maintain their body temperature and helped us bond. It also helped me with my milk production. Sometimes Eric would have one baby and I would have the other. My favorite time was when I could have both of them together on my chest. I never wanted it to end. I cannot tell you how much I loved Kangaroo Care. It helped me feel close to them and also made me feel useful.

Home Sweet Home??

As we got closer to my release date, I had such mixed emotions. We knew that the babies would be in the NICU most likely until close to their due date which was several weeks away. It was so nice to have my room just right upstairs from them. I got to see the babies as often as

Full Heart Empty Womb

I wanted. I could go down and see them in the middle of the night after I pumped. However, I was still so tired that I needed to be able to take breaks and rest. The NICU just had a hard rocking chair between their beds. It got pretty uncomfortable for me pretty quickly. I also could only stand for so long because I was so weak. It was nice to have a bed close by on which I could go lie down when I felt overwhelmed.

By this point I hadn't been home or slept in my bed in two months. I hadn't had a decent night's sleep in what seemed like forever. I longed for my quiet house with no beeps, intercoms, or sterile smell. I also hadn't done anything that I wanted to do to finish up their nursery. Yes, I was ready to see our little old house again.

On the day that I had to leave, I cried so hard when I kissed the babies goodbye. I knew for a while now that I would leave the hospital without my babies, but it still didn't make it any easier. I hadn't gone more than two to three hours at most without seeing them in the last few days. Now I was going to be a 45-minute car ride away.

I sat in my wheelchair waiting for Eric to pull up the minivan to the hospital entrance. I leaned my head back and breathed in the crisp fall Tennessee air for the first time in forever. He pulled up in my silver minivan and I smiled. On the way home, silent tears fell as I got farther and farther away from my babies. Then I looked up at the rolling hills and saw the beautiful leaves changing colors. Red, yellow, orange, and a few purple. My tears flowed faster. "I prayed that I would be able to go home and not miss the leaves change" I told Eric. I was thankful for another answered prayer no matter how small.

My sister, Amy, flew up from Texas to help me and see the babies. She had two little girls and I knew it wasn't an easy trip for her to make. I was so grateful she came. Amy had been one of my biggest prayer warriors over the last couple of years. If it were possible, I think her prayers alone had prayed Ethan and Ella into existence. Every year on their birthday she will put one of their pictures from the NICU on Facebook. I am so touched by the hordes of people that I have never met that comment about remembering praying for us! The power of prayer is awesome.

By then Eric had gone back to work, and it was so nice to have some company. I wasn't cleared to drive yet, so it was another blessing to have Amy join me each day on my hospital trips. We got into a routine with our hospital visits. I would get up early and go the hospital. Then I would go back to the house to rest for a few hours and return in the evening. Other times I would go a little later and have a marathon day. Either way it was exhausting.

Our New Normal

After about a week the babies were moved from the high level NICU to the "step down NICU". By then they were off their oxygen. Their main goals would be to learn how to eat on their own and get bigger. That wasn't going to be an easy task. We sure enjoyed the nicer surroundings though. They were in an actual crib instead of an incubator. The best part was that they were in a bed *together*. That provided me so much comfort to see them together again. Even when I wasn't able to be there, they would never be alone. The nurses even swaddled them together. They were a big double baby burrito!

Every day I would go and sit next to their beds. I would stare at the monitors that measured their heart rate, blood pressure, and oxygen levels. I would tap my foot to the steady beeps of the machines. Sometimes there would be a loud alarm beep and I would stop breathing. Usually it was when one of their sensors came loose. It took a while before I quit jumping each time I heard it. It was amazing to watch the nurses remain calm in the midst of constant alarms and over-emotional parents. Even when they needed to be alarmed because a baby had temporarily stopped breathing, they would react quickly, quietly, and unnoticeably to turn the lights back to green and the alarms back to mere beeps.

I loved to go at night because that was generally when they bathed them. Since they were still so little, the nurses had to be very careful about maintaining their body temperature. There was no baby tub. We got all of our supplies ready so that we could work quickly. We had several washcloths that we soaked in very warm water and lathered up with baby soap. We wet several others with just warm water. The babies were swaddled up and we unwrapped one body part at a time and quickly washed, dried, and covered them up.

As we bathed the babies, the nurses changed the sheets on their beds. My mom had made several blankets for each of the babies. I loved that the NICU nurses were so good about covering their bed and swaddling them in their Mimi blankets. It made the sterile NICU feel a little bit more like home. They also put them in some of the sleepers that we brought from home. Even the preemie outfits swallowed them but we made them work.

Hello. I am a Cow.

I met with a lactation consultant to try to learn how I could nurse the babies. I wasn't ready to give up on being able to breastfeed yet. The fact that breast milk was best for them was hammered into my head. If providing them with breast milk was going to help them get stronger, then by gosh I was going to do it. We attempted to nurse a few times. They just couldn't do it. They were too weak and it wore them out. It wore me out, too. I was so nervous that I was trying to get them to do too much. I would watch the clock and think that the longer we tried the longer it would be until they got that much needed nourishment in their little bellies. It was incredibly stressful for me. Not at all what I imagined the nursing experience to be.

I finally got to the point where I just told the lactation consultant that we weren't going to try to nurse anymore until they were older. I would continue to pump and just bottle feed them. She encouraged me to take several supplements and vitamins to help boost my milk production. They weren't always going to be eating just one ounce at a time. I needed to be ready to meet their needs. She also told me to start pumping every two hours during the daytime hours. I nodded energetically. Whatever I could do to help my babies, I was ready to do.

When I was at the hospital, I would time my pumping so that it was right before they ate so they could have fresh milk. When I pumped at home, I would freeze the milk to be used later. Before long our entire freezer was full of breast milk. There was no room for even a Hot Pocket. But that didn't matter because we were never home to eat anyway!

At first, when I pumped at night, I needed Eric's help. It was so hard for me to go from lying down to sitting up because of my C-section. Eric would help me get into a comfortable position and bring me my breast pump. I would watch TV for 20 minutes while I pumped and Eric would take a catnap. I would wake him up and he would take the pump back to wash and sterilize it for the next time. We would do it all over again two and a half hours later. Talk about exhausting.

Eventually I learned that I had to roll on to my side and use my arms to push me up so that I didn't use any of my abdominal muscles. I had healed enough that I could get around pretty well on my own. I encouraged him to sleep through it since he had to work the next day.

I invested in a double pump. I even got this contraption to hold it for me so I could just sit back and let it do its job. Best money I ever spent. It was exhausting pumping in the middle of the night and every little bit helped. I always had to watch TV to help pass the time more quickly. In late October there was never a shortage of good scary movies to watch in the middle of the night, which I loved. One night I pumped during various parts of all the *Halloween* movies. When Eric got up the next morning, he begged me to not watch scary movies anymore. "I had nightmares and all I could hear was that horrible

Full Heart Empty Womb

Michael Myers theme music in my head all night (da-da da-da da-da na-na)!!"

After a while, the long days at the NICU and lack of solid sleep took their toll on me. One day when Dr. Blake came by to see the babies, I had a breakdown with her. She was so calm and caring with me. She encouraged me to take better care of myself so that I could be ready to take care of the babies when they went home. She also encouraged me to take a night off from the pumping so that I could get some solid sleep. Since the day they were born, I had not slept more than a couple of hours at a time.

I was so grateful to hear those words from her. I needed to hear that from her. I began to see the tiny silver lining around the babies' NICU stay. My body had been through hell and back. I had a hard enough time getting through the day as it was. At least now I had a lot of support from all the nurses and doctors taking care of Ethan and Ella. I had to try to be better about letting myself heal so I could be ready to take care of them when they came home.

That night I went to bed and did not set my alarm. It was a glorious feeling. I slept hard. I slept well. I slept for a solid eight hours without waking up which is unheard of for me. When I woke though, I was very engorged from missing three pumping sessions. It hurt so bad that I cried. I immediately set up the pump to get some relief. I was so engorged that it was hard to even pump so I took a really hot shower to help. I pumped. And pumped. I spent all day pumping to try to get relief from my precious night's sleep.

I appreciated that night of sleep. But needless to say, I never did it again. I really felt that if I was awake, then I needed to be by their bedside. I even felt guilty when I slept and that wasn't very much. But I did try to heed my doctor's advice and allow myself time to rest and heal.

One Month and Counting….

After about a month in the NICU, it became clear that the babies needed a little more help. We were at a standstill. They were gaining weight and had not had any apnea episodes in a while. However, the poor babies just couldn't get the hang of taking a bottle. They didn't have the coordination to drink a bottle, swallow, and continue breathing. They would also often fall asleep when we gave them their tiny bottles. If they still had not finished their ounce of milk after a while, we would have to put it through their feeding tubes so they wouldn't burn too many calories overexerting themselves.

In order for them to be released they had to be able to take a full bottle consistently over a few days. We wouldn't have a feeding tube to fall back on at home! We got so excited when they finally got a whole bottle down. Then with the next bottle they were hardly able to drink any of it. It was frustrating. We were so ready to have our babies home with us.

The neonatologists suggested that we allow Ethan and Ella to have a transfusion to help them gain strength. My mom highly encouraged it. Her mom, Mema, had had one once when she was really weak in the hospital and it really helped her gain the needed strength. The doctors assured us that it was safe. They went through all of the procedures that they have in place to make sure the blood is safe. We agreed to let them have the transfusion and were hopeful that this would be what they needed to turn the corner.

The transfusion worked wonders for them. Their color improved. They were more alert. They were finally able to take an entire bottle more consistently. Because they were doing so much better, the nurses told me that I could hold the babies more.

Before now, I would sit by their crib all day. I would anxiously wait until I was able to feed them their bottles or do Kangaroo Care just so I could hold my babies. I cannot tell you the anxiety I felt about whether or not they were going to be able to bond with me because of our lack of physical contact. The nurses assured me that it wouldn't be a problem but I couldn't help but worry. Most newborns live from lap to lap in constant contact with their Mommy and Daddy. We were lucky if we got an hour a day. We were not allowed to hold them more than that for fear that it would interrupt their much needed sleep.

But now I had the green light. It was fantastic. I came into the NICU ready to catch up on all the loving that I had missed out on the last four weeks. I would sit in my hard rocking chair and the nurses would help put both Ethan and Ella in my arms. My eyes teared up with love and gratitude. I would never take this for granted. I kissed their tiny heads, whispered "I love you", and sang a song to them about how "Mommy Loves You". I couldn't wait to come back with Eric that night and we could both rock babies all night. We would finally be a normal family…except we were in a NICU.

Over the next couple of weeks Ethan and Ella continued to get stronger. They started to drink more milk and were able to take more and more bottles without any assistance. It was exciting but nerve wracking at the same time. All it took was one apnea episode or one missed bottle and we were back to square one.

I prayed that they continued to do well. I also prayed that Ethan and Ella stayed on the same pattern. It broke my heart to think about one of them going home and the other staying even one more day. It always warmed my heart to think that they were snuggled up together in bed when I wasn't there. They weren't ever by themselves. It would make me so sad to have them separated. It would also be very difficult on me logistically to have one in the NICU and one at home. Once a baby leaves the NICU, they cannot come back. The NICU cannot risk any outside infection coming into the unit. The situation would mean I would need to get my mom or mother-in-law to come and stay with the baby at home. They would happily agree, of course. But it would make me feel torn. At the NICU I got to spend time with both of my babies.

I tried to stay positive and I excitedly put the finishing touches on their nursery so it was ready for their arrival. I washed tiny clothes and put them in the drawers. I stocked up on itty bitty diapers. I took their car seats to the fire department to get them installed properly.

Home Sweet Home!!

On the day before Thanksgiving, five weeks and one day after they entered this world, Ethan and Ella finally got to come home. We were ecstatic and a little scared. It was a blessing that we got to work alongside the nurses for the last several weeks and learned how to do everything from the pros. However, we also had the comfort of monitors that assured us that they were breathing, their oxygen level was right, and their blood pressure was where it needed to be.

Eric pulled our new minivan up to the front of the hospital to pick us up. It probably took us 20 minutes to get them loaded in properly. I sat in the back with them for the ride home talking and singing to them the whole way.

As soon as we got home, we introduced them to Majors. He was not very impressed. I am sure he thought, "These little things are what you left me for?" He was still getting over his hurt feelings about being shipped to my parents' house in Kentucky while I was in the hospital!

We carefully unloaded them from their car seats and walked them up to their nursery. We laid them in their crib together and smiled down at them. Then we looked at each other as if to say, "Okay. Now what??" They promptly started to fuss and that kicked us into gear.

Full House

We had one night of just the four of us at home. The next day my parents and my sister's family all came to our house to spend Thanksgiving. I would like to say it was because they wanted to spend Thanksgiving with me, but I think they had two other very good reasons.

I will be honest. I don't remember much about their first Thanksgiving. It was chaotic. It was loud. It was full of love. There was no shortage of people who were ready to feed or rock a baby.

Flying By the Seat of Our Pants

When everyone left, Eric and I had to establish our own routine. There was a lot of trial and error. At first we had them set up in a bassinet in our room. I couldn't have them close enough to me. Then we discovered that Ella was quite a noisy sleeper so the bassinet got farther and farther away from us. Finally the last step was to move the pack-n-play into our bathroom and even turn on the fan. You could say we had gotten over our dependency on the monitors from the NICU!

After about a week we decided to finally just move them upstairs into their crib. It only took one night before we moved upstairs with them. Some nights I was so tired that I just laid down on the floor in their nursery. Most nights Eric and I slept on a combination twin-trundle bed that was in my home office. We would wake up startled from the crying and whoever was in the trundle usually got pounced on.

It was such a crazy exhausting time. I was still pumping every three hours. Added to that I was feeding the babies every three hours. So that meant that I got roughly an hour and a half of sleep at a time.

We tried to take shifts feeding the babies so the other could sleep but it just didn't work. They required too much help when taking a bottle. They would still fall asleep while taking the bottle so we had to try to keep them awake. You couldn't do that if your attention was divided between the two babies. Even with just one of the babies, it still took about 30 to 45 minutes for them to drink most of their bottle. We got into the routine of watching 24 reruns at each feeding. Jack Bauer got us through a lot of nights!

I admit I was a bit of an obsessed new mama. I continued to follow the NICU orders to the letter once we got home. Before every bottle I took their temperature, changed their diaper, and recorded it on an Excel spreadsheet. Yes another spreadsheet. I even made grandparents do it. I can only imagine the conversations that they had on the way home from our house about how crazy I was. I did this routine for a full two months at home until the pediatrician told me I didn't have to do that. I can only imagine the conversation he had with his nurses after I left!

I was fortunate to have my mother-in-law come and help me sometimes. My parents visited as often as they could. They were building a home for their retirement nearby and would move in a few months. They helped me keep my sanity and enabled me to just get to the grocery store.

We were running on Diet Coke, prayers, and fumes. When I look back at how little sleep we got and still functioned, I am amazed. I don't think I could do it now.

Whatsa Masta What?

I was continuing my one-woman milk factory efforts. I felt pressure to continue to increase my milk production. "They will be drinking big bottles before you know it!" the lactation consultants hammered into my head.

I started to get a pretty painful lump in one breast. I would pump more and try to massage it out but it never seemed to work. It got to the point where it brought me to tears with even the gentlest touch. Of course I called my go-to nurse, Kristen, for advice. She was also my breastfeeding/pumping expert. She told me that she thought I had mastitis and asked if I felt bad or was running a fever. What?? Of course I feel bad! I never get to sleep. I thought this whirlwind is just what having newborn twins feels like! After her prodding, I got an immediate appointment with Dr. Blake.

You know that when you go to the doctor and she asks her nurse to come and 'take a look at this', it is not a good sign. Apparently I had mastitis pretty badly. And in true Steph fashion, I kicked it up a notch and got an abscess. My infection was so severe that I was close to hospitalization for IV antibiotics. Thank God I didn't have to do that because separation from my babies would have been horrible.

However, I did have to go to a breast specialist and have the abscess drained. Yes, it was every bit as horrible and painful as you can imagine. I had to go back repeatedly to have it drained and redressed until it healed.

I also had to stop pumping immediately. It was a blessing and a curse. I was sad that I couldn't provide the babies breast milk anymore; I was so glad that we had such a stockpile of it in our freezer! But I feel like it was a blessing because this event took it out of my hands. God knew that I would pump indefinitely because I wanted what I was told was best for my babies. Now I had permission - no, orders - to take care of myself. I instantly got a few more hours of desperately needed sleep each day!

Our New Normal

Since the babies came home right at the beginning of cold and flu season, we hung out at home most of the time. I had decided to resign from my job and be a stay at home mom. It was the best decision I ever made. I was extremely grateful that Eric saw the value of my staying home with the babies. Sure the expense of twice the childcare factored into it but it was just the simple fact that I didn't want to be anywhere but with my two sweet babies. We had fought hard enough for them. I wasn't going to miss one single minute.

And I didn't miss a single minute. We were strongly encouraged to not get out in public much because they could get sick so easily. I had no problem following those orders. I knew the slightest cold could mean the worst for them, and they could end up back in the hospital.

Not to mention the fact that the logistics of getting two babies out of the house made my head hurt. Their strict bottle schedule meant that I would either have to pack a bottle and be ready to feed them while out or I was limited to very short excursions. Between the packing up and stress of having them out, I was ready for a nap or a drink by the time I got home. I often chose the easy path and stayed home. Those poor babies didn't really leave the house until they were six months old!

We were so blessed. The babies continued to grow and thrive. They were right on target with their development by their adjusted age. The adjusted age was what their age would be if they had been born on their due date. For Ethan and Ella that meant that they had a two month delay for most of their milestones. The only milestone they came close to missing was walking. They both literally started walking the day before they would have been considered behind. They started walking just in time for things to get a little more interesting…

Chapter Five – Miracle High

Life can be a series of highs and lows. My life has certainly been a testament to that. Met and married my wonderful husband Eric – High. Tried to conceive for a couple of years, failed fertility treatments, surgery – Low. Successfully got pregnant through IVF – HUGE High! High risk pregnancy that left me on bed rest for what felt like most of my pregnancy – Low. Delivering premature but healthy twins – High/Low. Five weeks and one day of being separated from them in the NICU – Low.

I could go on and on. I want to share with you one of my favorite Highs. He is my little Miracle High. Eric and I were told that there was absolutely no way that we could conceive naturally. For that reason we went through IVF to conceive Ethan and Ella. I have no doubt that it was, indeed, a fact. As I said this is a *Miracle* High.

January 2008

I woke up just like the day before. I had no idea that this morning would change all of our lives so much! Eric was getting ready for work and I was lying in bed watching Sports Center (his choice, not mine). I remembered that I needed to call in a prescription that day. Before I could get it, I had to take a pregnancy test. My cycle was running way too long and I needed to get on progesterone to get me back on track. I always thought this was a funny thing for me, of all people, to have to do. I mean, we know I can't get pregnant. On top of that, I went back on birth control after I had Ethan and Ella. I was simply taking it for convenience sake. Eric and I often laughed about what money we wasted on all those birth control pills early in our marriage. So off I went to pee on my little stick. I unloaded the dishwasher, sat down, and watched TV for a minute. Should I get the kids up? Oh no wait…better go check the test and get that out of the way.

Full Heart Empty Womb

I walked into the guest bath and looked at the test on the sink. Double take...were those TWO lines? Huh? I must be seeing things. I heard Eric say something so I threw the hand towel over the test and jumped back in bed. Eric said, "Why do you look so weird?" I was still in shock so I said, "Just tired." He went back to the closet to finish getting dressed and I ran back to the bathroom for a second look. Yes. Definitely two lines. How did this happen??? I mean I know how it happens for most, but not us! We were told that we *couldn't* get pregnant on our own. Holy cow. Eric's birthday was the next day. Boy, could I have fun with this!!! I ran upstairs to get the babies up and whispered my secret in their tiny ears. I was pretty sure they smiled.

Thankfully Eric left shortly after that. I am told later that I am in MAJOR trouble for letting him go to work because he would have called in sick. Whoops. I quickly called my mom, my sister, and Kristen. Kristen, my personal OB nurse, reassured me that the home tests are pretty accurate. Even so, I had my mom come over so I could get an official blood test at the doctor's office. I still didn't believe it. I went and looked at the home test again. Still two lines! When I called Dr. Blake's office to get the test they acted like I was crazy. "Mrs. Greer, we usually don't do blood tests if you have a positive home test." I replied, "I know, but I don't believe it. When can I come in?" I went in immediately, got my blood drawn, and paid to have the results to me stat.

I cried and prayed on the whole way home from the doctor's office. I was smiling ear to ear and laughing as I praised God. I am sure anyone who passed by me on the road thought I was crazy. And I was. Crazy happy. I couldn't believe God's blessing on us. How could this be? It took so much for us to get pregnant with Ethan and Ella. Nothing had changed with us. We were still infertile. I mean, I was on BIRTH CONTROL too! This was really a miracle straight from above.

All day I avoided calls from Eric and his sister, Amy. How in the world could I play this one off? I couldn't even sit down I was so excited! I finally got the "official positive" test results from the doctor. Hallelujah!

Full Heart Empty Womb

Praise God!! I checked the home test one more time and finally threw it in the trash.

Now how in the world would I give Eric the total shock of his lifetime??? The way we found out we were pregnant with Ethan and Ella was so impersonal. We called into a voicemail box and listened to a stranger tell us the good news. Not that we minded one bit. We were finally pregnant!!

I decided I would get the kids Big Brother and Big Sister t-shirts, take their pictures in it, frame it, and give it to Eric for his birthday. Well I am not sure how many of you have tried to get a 16-month old kid to stand still so you can get a good picture of him. Now throw in a second child. It isn't possible. Just take it from me. So I decided the next best thing was to just wrap up the shirts and let Eric open those.

We waited on pins and needles until Eric got home. Of course since we were anxiously awaiting him, he didn't get home until after 7. After the kids' bath, Eric read them a story, and then they just had to give their Daddy an early birthday present. He didn't know it, but I recorded the whole thing. This was the experience that we always dreamed about having - just the pure joy of getting pregnant with no drama!

Eric sat in the rocking chair in the babies' room with both of them on his lap. I told him that we were too excited to wait and we just had to give him his present that night. He wasn't surprised. I was the worst at keeping secrets! I handed him his present, and he took his sweet, precious time unwrapping it.

When he finally opened the box that held the Big Brother and Big Sister t-shirts, he tried unsuccessfully to hide his confusion. "Oh wow," he said to the babies with as much enthusiasm as he could pretend to have. "What do we have here?" He pulled out Ethan's shirt first. "So you got a big brother shirt because you are the oldest. And you Sissy are the big sister because you are big. HA!!" He thought he made a really funny joke because at the time Ella was bigger than

Ethan. He was still completely CLUELESS. I shouldn't have given him a hard time. We were told it was impossible....

Eric looked up at me trying to look really excited about getting a couple of baby t-shirts. Still clueless. I had to put him out of his misery. "That is not the only reason why, Eric" I said to him and gave it a second to sink in.

He continued to look at me blankly, then looked back down to the shirts. I said, "I'm pregnant!!" His head snapped right back up and he immediately started to cry. The four of us sat in our little rocking chair and cried and praised God for what seemed like forever.

We basked in our miracle and the glimpse of what getting pregnant "normally" was. The other crazy part was that my due date was Ethan and Ella's second birthday! Exactly two years to the day!

We had a big family birthday party with our parents and Eric's sister's family a couple of days later. We told them they had to see this video of what the kids gave Eric for his birthday. It was hysterical to watch their reactions. The ladies immediately got it and started crying and hugging. The guys all had lost looks for a minute before it sunk in. It was the best birthday ever.

Pregnancy Guilt

For a while I felt like I was just pretending I was pregnant. It didn't feel real. Really, I wasn't supposed to be able to get pregnant on my own. It didn't take long for me to go from happiness to feeling guilty. Of course I was *over the moon* that I was pregnant! But I couldn't help but think about the frozen embryos that we had in storage. In fact we had just paid for our first year of storage for them not long ago. Over the past year, we had thought about them and our plans for them often. We were overwhelmed new parents of twins, so we were thinking about going back for a frozen embryo transfer in two or three years. I knew that I couldn't be a good mom to any more children than the two I had then!

The guilt I felt is kind of hard to understand. I felt like we had a responsibility to those embryos first. Were we irresponsible? Should we have been more careful to not get pregnant before we had an opportunity to try to get pregnant with our frozen embryos?

Seriously. I was infertile. It took pretty much the maximum intervention there is in the infertility world to get me pregnant. I was on birth control. We had twins that hardly slept, so there was little activity in *our* bedroom. This was borderline immaculate conception! This was a true, honest to God miracle. If it were not for God's direct intervention, I would not be pregnant. God made what was completely impossible possible in my infertile body.

No, this guilt was 100% from Satan who was trying to take this gift - this pure God given joy - away from me. And I was letting him! I can't wait to get to Heaven and be able to talk to God and see why he chose to bless me with the pregnancy and the timing of it. Was it a blessing for being faithful throughout my pregnancy with Ethan and Ella? Or was it a 'pay it forward' for the pain I would have several years down the road? Regardless, I had to just accept this miracle and be thankful. Once I put the guilt to rest, that was an easy thing to do!

Sick and Tired

I felt the pregnancy symptoms sooner this go around. I felt nauseous but never got sick. I desperately wanted to just throw up so I would feel better. I just walked around feeling sick with a baggie of saltines in my hands. Except this time I had two little greedy kids that liked to steal all my crackers!!

I was also incredibly tired. I was told by Eric, my family, and my doctor to rest when the babies did. I did my best but it was difficult.

Ethan and Ella were almost 18 months old and into *everything*. They had just gotten used to walking and were determined to never sit down again which kind of made it difficult for me to sit.

We spent a small fortune on baby gates trying to keep them contained and safe. We even bought a "play yard" that was a series of interlocking plastic gates that made a jumbo playpen. It was a sanity saver for me. I had somewhere I could put the babies and pee (which I was doing often) and not be afraid of them falling down the stairs. We could buy extensions to make it bigger. Eventually we bought enough that it took up most of our playroom. I could lie down inside of it and the babies would climb and play all over my lazy bones.

Reality Check

When I was eight weeks along, I woke up and was spotting. I called Dr. Blake in a panic. She assured me that spotting is normal for some pregnant women. The only thing that I could do was to take it easy. I had heard that spotting happened with many of my friends. Why don't they just go ahead and warn you of that from the get go? I felt a little better because it was nothing like the hemorrhage that I had when I was pregnant with Ethan and Ella. However, you never feel at all at ease when you are bleeding and pregnant.

My sister, Amy, and her girls were up visiting for their Spring Break at the time. We canceled our plans for the day and just hung out together so I could lie on the couch. Even though I continued to have pregnancy symptoms, I didn't feel better until I went to the doctor and heard the heartbeat with my own ears.

We talked with Dr. Blake about what safety measures we needed to take given all of the pregnancy complications I had before. She didn't believe it was an absolute certainty that I would have any complications this time. The complications from my previous pregnancy could have been because I was carrying twins. We were sure that I was pregnant with a singleton this time.

We discussed the possibility of my getting a cervical cerclage. A cerclage is a procedure to stitch a woman's cervix closed during pregnancy to help prevent miscarriage. As with any medical procedure, a cerclage has risks, too. The issue with my cervix was that it shortened. I never dilated until the day I delivered Ethan and Ella. We decided that a cerclage would not address the problems that I had with my cervix.

I was given the order to rest as much as I could. I was not supposed to pick up the babies if I could help it. I would also go to the high-risk doctors again so that they could monitor me closely given my history of preterm labor.

Pregnant with One Year Old Twins in Tow

Always the good patient, I followed the doctor's orders to the best of my ability. I felt the weight of the world on my shoulders. I had to do everything that I could to minimize any chance of me going into premature labor again. The idea of being hospitalized and away from my babies was more than I could even bear to think about. I spent countless hours crying from thinking about the possibility.

Fortunately my mom and mother-in-law were happy to come and help occasionally. Ethan and Ella were always happy to bribe them with their sweet kisses. I was so grateful. The not-so-simple task of just taking them to the grocery store with me had turned into the impossible. Even if we could muddle through them climbing into the van and up to their car seats by themselves, there was no way I could get them in a grocery cart without picking them up! I knew I wasn't forbidden from picking them up yet, but I had to do everything I could to minimize how much I did.

Once I started to show, the few times I did go out with them I got several double-takes. Ethan and Ella were still very small for their age so they probably didn't even look to be a year old. I remember distinctly a trip to Costco when I had my feelings hurt by a stranger. A lady and her husband walked by me and did an exaggerated double-take. Then she said quite loudly, "Can you *believe* that?? She has twins that little and she is already having another one." She sounded absolutely disgusted. She was disgusted by my joy. My miracles.

Now I don't presume to know her history or where her hatred came from. Perhaps she assumed that I was irresponsible and that I didn't know the whole concept of "birth control". I think these first four chapters establish that it was not the case. Perhaps she thought her hard earned tax dollars were "helping me take care of the kids I kept having". Eric worked hard every day to provide for us. I clipped every coupon I could find to help save our hard earned money. Perhaps she too was infertile and was hurt and bitter by seeing any pregnant woman let alone one who already had twins. Regardless, it was a good reminder to me that you never know what a stranger is going through and you should never rush to judgment.

Pins and Needles

I tried to enjoy my pregnancy, and I did for the most part. However, I always had worry and anxiety waiting in the wings to overshadow my joy. I am ashamed that I let it get the best of me more often than not. I worried about overdoing it during the day. I tried to take it easy but I could only do that so much with two very active toddlers that were excited about discovering every little detail. I felt guilty because I didn't take my kids to all the fun activities that it seemed that everyone else was doing. Going to story time at the library. Mommy and Me classes. Even just going to the park. On the days that I did venture out with them, I would come home beyond exhausted and riddled with guilt. I felt like I couldn't win. We spent most days hanging out in our play yard singing songs and reading books over and over. Now I can look back and see that was all in the world they needed.

If I were to even think about our frozen embryos, I would start to panic. How did I get from "Dear Lord, please let me have a baby!" to "Dear Lord, how many babies am I going to have?" I was exhausted with two babies and trying to figure out how I was going to raise a third. We would have to wait a while before we could even think about doing an embryo transfer, for sure.

At one point, when we went for an ultrasound, they detected a heart murmur in the baby. We were assured that it was normal and would most likely resolve itself before I gave birth. They would just keep an even closer eye on me for the rest of the pregnancy. I was frustrated that they had yet another cause for concern. However, I was comforted that they were going to watch me more closely. I would have even more ultrasounds. I was so afraid I was going to go into premature labor again and not know it.

Peanut

The next ultrasound we went to was when they could determine the sex of the baby. I was adamant that we were not going to find out. Why did we need to? We had saved all of Ethan and Ella's stuff so we were set with clothes no matter if it was a boy or a girl. I wanted to make this pregnancy as much fun as possible. The idea of the sex being a surprise was invigorating to me.

I was so proud when we made it through the whole ultrasound without asking. When the ultrasound tech told us she was going to write down the sex and put it in a sealed envelope, I told her to not even bother with it. Eric knowingly nodded and slipped the envelope in his back pocket.

Full Heart Empty Womb

I made it a full two weeks before I broke down and opened it. It all came down to paint. Ethan and Ella's nursery had been gender neutral. I wanted to be able to have a pretty pink or baby blue nursery for once! I decided it would be the perfect birthday present for me to be able to go buy some paint!

I also hated calling the baby 'it'. We had adopted the nickname, "Peanut," for the baby but inevitably the baby was still called 'it' sometimes. That irked me to no end. The bottom line was that I just wanted to know. I wanted to be able to imagine my sweet baby and give Peanut a name so I could sing to him or her. And so I looked as Eric was driving down the road because I couldn't wait another moment once I got Eric's blessing to look. We found out I was going to have another sweet boy!

The further along I got, the more prepared I was for the bottom to fall out at any minute. The first half of my pregnancy I was worried about premature labor but I didn't think it was anything imminent. As I progressed in my pregnancy, I started to worry about the reality that I could start going into premature labor at any time.

By the time I was in my third trimester, I would go to my weekly ultrasounds with a packed bag expecting to be admitted that day. I would cry the whole morning as I got ready for my big outing that week. I would kiss Ethan and Ella's heads like it was the last time I would see them for a while because I believed it was.

I had an elaborate plan in place with Eric and my mom. My mom was generally who would stay with the babies while I went to the ultrasound. Mom would pack a bag too sometimes just in case she needed to stay if I went into the hospital. I had so many doctor appointments that I discouraged Eric from coming so he wouldn't miss too much work. He had his phone close by when I was there.

Week after week we did this routine. It kind of felt like Groundhog Day. Fortunately, every week my cervix held strong, and there were no contractions. By the time I made it through the hot Tennessee summer,

I finally figured out that we may be out of the woods. For ten long weeks, I kissed my babies goodbye thinking that surely this was the week that I would be admitted to the hospital.

We finally reached the point that we got to actually schedule the C-section. I didn't want to go all the way to my due date since it was Ethan and Ella's second birthday. The soonest they would schedule it was a week before. After all this anxiety and worry, we could actually look at the due date like most couples and visualize when our son was going to be born!

Eric's Chili

Like most Saturdays in the fall, we were enjoying a day of football. Rather, Eric was enjoying a Saturday of football, and I was enjoying a little bit here and there between taking care of the babies. I didn't mind though. Tennessee football is his passion. He works like a dog all week to provide for us, so I am happy for him to have at least one day to relax.

And he doesn't entirely relax. Eric really is the best cook ever. He loves to grill and does it wonderfully. He also loves to make chili. He has very specific rules about when you are "allowed" to make chili. It has to be October or after. You can't have chili in September! AND it has to be less than 70 degrees. Hey, I don't make the rules (or the chili). I just enjoy it when it is made. And enjoy it I did. I had a chili dog with a side of chili cheese Fritos and enjoyed every last bite. I may have even had a little baby bowl of just plain chili. I went to bed with a full belly and a smile on my face.

I woke up around four a.m. because my stomach felt odd. I was up and down for the rest of the night because I just felt off. I complained to Eric a bit about how his chili upset my stomach. I was not about to make a big deal about it though. Between my doctor appointments and Sunday church, those were the only times I got to leave the house!

And since I was about to have a baby in a week, I wasn't even going to be doing that much longer.

I smiled through my discomfort as we drove to church. I shifted and grimaced as I sat in my Sunday school class. After a few stomach cramps I realized that these "cramps" were coming actually quite regularly. Oh my. I leaned over to Eric and said, "Hey don't panic, but I am pretty sure I have been having contractions for like the last six hours. As soon as Howard finishes the prayer we need to bust a move." His eyes went as wide as saucers.

As soon as our teacher, Howard, said "Amen" Eric grabbed my hand and we flew out the door. We ran through the preschool hallway and grabbed Ethan and Ella. As we drove home, I called my mom and asked her and my dad to come to the house. "We are having a baby today!" I called my sister to tell her. She laughed and cried and said, "I asked my class to pray that you would have Peanut a little early so he would be here when we came to visit!" Apparently Amy's prayers are pretty potent!

We got home and put the babies right in their highchairs. Eric got busy putting some lunch together for them while I got my bag and everything ready to head to the hospital. My parents sailed in just in time for us to hop back in the van and head to the hospital.

I giggled from excited anticipation and groaned from painful contractions the whole way to the hospital. I couldn't believe how painful the contractions were. I couldn't talk and could hardly breathe in the midst of one. How in the world was I having contractions continually with Ethan and Ella and never felt one? It still baffles me to this day.

When we got to the hospital I was ushered into a room per Dr. Blake's orders. She was off this day but one of her colleagues was going to perform the C-section. I had met this doctor during my time in the hospital with Ethan and Ella and liked her very much. She was also my mom's gynecologist so I felt like I was in good hands.

Full Heart Empty Womb

Unfortunately, I wasn't the only person who decided to have a baby on that Sunday afternoon, so she couldn't come right to me. The nurses told me that they could go ahead and administer pain meds, but I wanted to wait until they absolutely had to. For some reason I was paranoid that they would wear off before I really needed them! So I laid on my side in my bed and watched the clock and timed my contractions. I never did any child birthing classes because I knew that I was going to have a C-section. At that time I sure wished that I knew some good breathing techniques to help me deal with the pain!

Baby Matthew

I was certainly ready when they said it was time to take me back to the operating room. I was just so excited to meet my little Peanut. It was such a different experience from the last time. Everything was so calm and happy. I was alert and aware of everything that was going on. I didn't look or feel like I had come straight from "Night of the Living Dead" like I did with Ethan and Ella.

The doctor and nurses worked quickly and efficiently and before I knew it I heard the cry of Matthew Kenneth Greer. They held him up to show me before they cleaned him up. I saw a mess of dark brown hair and perfect pink skin and tears sprang to my eyes. They cleaned him up quickly, swaddled him, and gave Matthew to a smiling Eric.

Eric brought him over to me and I got to *hold* and kiss my sweet baby immediately. No waiting for 24 hours. I got to hold and cherish my sweet boy right then. I was so grateful. He opened his eyes and looked directly into mine. We shared the same brown eyes. I saw the recognition immediately. He knew I was his Mommy. Oh, what an unexpected blessing from God!

Eric went with the nurses to get Matthew cleaned up while they finished with me. The doctor confirmed that I wanted my tubes tied. I said, "Yes. Real tight please." I knew that since I was infertile it wasn't really necessary. But given the guilt that I had been dealing with about our frozen embryos, it was entirely necessary in my mind.

Our stay in the hospital was so *normal*. It seemed like forever before they brought Matthew to me, but it really wasn't. Five minutes would have been too long. I wanted to snuggle my baby! They brought him to me and just told me to let them know if we wanted them to come get him and take him to the nursery. "Wait – you mean we get to just have our baby here with us for as long as we want? We can just *hold* our baby and no one is going to tell us that he needs to be back in his bed so he isn't overstimulated??" This concept was completely foreign to us. And completely awesome!

I desperately wanted to be able to breastfeed Matthew. It was something that I accepted I couldn't do with Ethan and Ella but that I always wished I could. With very little help Matthew was able to latch on and nurse. I was so excited. I could have nursed him all day while staring at his sweet, perfect face and holding his precious little feet. At times it felt like I did do it all day!

My father-in-law, Brent, and mother-in-law, Sarah, came into town to help watch Ethan and Ella. They took turns with my parents so that they could come and see Matthew. I think that getting to experience a "normal" childbirth was pretty neat for Brent and Sarah too. Of all of their six grandchildren, Matthew was the only one that was not immediately admitted to the NICU. My sister-in-law, Amy, had triplets prematurely, too. It was nice for everyone to be able to hold and love on Matthew immediately. The only problem was that there was only one of him so we had to take turns!

We decided to wait until the next day before Ethan and Ella came to meet their new little brother. Ethan and Ella came in wearing the same t-shirts that we wrapped up for Daddy nine months before. They were happy to see Eric and me, but were more interested in the hospital bed and TV. When we introduced them to Baby Matthew they were a little unimpressed. When we showed them that Baby Matthew got them each a little gift, he grew on them a little.

I am not going to lie. I thoroughly loved every day that I stayed in the hospital. My only job was to heal and snuggle my baby. I didn't have to cook for anyone. I didn't have to clean up anything. I didn't have to jump up as soon as I sat down to get this or get that. I could just lie in my bed and enjoy being a mom. I so appreciated having the opportunity to see what most women go through when they have a baby.

All that being said, I desperately missed Ethan and Ella and was ready to go home and have all my babies under one roof! I was grateful that I got a lot of help from our parents. I don't know what I would have done without their support. My sister also came into town. Her prayers worked! I am so happy that she was able to be there so soon after my babies were born. She lives all the way in Texas, so it is a blessing that the timing worked out.

Another New Normal

We were officially outnumbered by three kids under two. Our life was crazy chaos and it was wonderful. Matthew was such a good baby. He pretty much just ate and slept until he was six weeks old. Then he got colic and life got pretty hairy. He screamed from about 5:00 at night until 10:00 at night. As difficult as having twins was, having a colicky baby could rival that any day.

He would start up about the time that I was trying to feed Ethan and Ella. I would walk and bounce Matthew as I was preparing their supper. Eric would usually get home as I was finishing dinner through a stream of tears. Eric would grab Matthew and walk and bounce him. Sometimes he could go in the bathroom with the fan going and that would calm him down a bit. After we put Ethan and Ella down for bed, we would lock ourselves in our room with a screaming Matthew trying to keep him from waking them. We took turns walking and bouncing him. We probably walked 10 miles each night in a circuit around our bed.

Since Matthew was born at the beginning of cold and flu season, we lived like hermits for yet another winter. It was fine by me though because the idea of my taking all three of them out made me very nervous. I finally got the nerve to take them out in the spring. I put Ethan and Ella in a double stroller and strapped Matthew in a Baby Bjorn on my chest. It was exhausting, but I felt empowered. I felt strong and confident that I could do this.

Feeling confident, not too long after that I went to the grocery store with all of them. I had to leave my cart in the middle of the aisle because one of the kids started to have a meltdown. I didn't have enough hands or sanity to deal with it.

There were many days that ended in tears from me. I wondered why God thought I could handle this stress. I never thought there was enough of me to go around. Have I held each of the babies enough today? Have I given each of them enough attention? If one of them was having a bad day, I felt guilty that I was neglecting the others. It was a horrible feeling. I never felt like I measured up.

Don't get me wrong. I would not trade one single second. However, the guilt that a mother can feel is pretty powerful. I think it is amplified if you suffer from infertility before you become a mother. It is what you wanted, you shouldn't be overwhelmed by it! Never mind the guilt that a woman feels when she runs out of steam at the end of the day from being a Mommy then has no energy to be a wife too.

Eric was always so patient and supportive of me. He worked very long hours that got him home many nights after the kids went to bed. He did this so that he could provide for our family and so that I could stay home with the kids. Although with three little ones now, I would have to get a very well-paying job to make it even financially reasonable for me to go back to work. But as stressful as life was, I wouldn't have had it any other way.

A Big Decision

Every day I would think about our four frozen embryos. Sometimes it was a quick thought that I dismissed because my mind couldn't even go there. Other times it was a long, tear filled prayer. I was getting better at juggling three kids, but it was still so hard. I never felt like I quite measured up.

The idea about being a mother to more than three children was overwhelming to me. Could I be a good mommy to more kids? Is there enough of me to go around? Can I be the kind of mommy that I want to be? I am an affectionate person. I loved to hug and kiss my babies all day long. I loved to have them sit on my lap and read them a book. I kissed their little heads with every turn of the page.

With three children, I don't get to do that as often as I would like. There is so much more to being a mommy than loving them. There are meals to make, laundry to do, rooms to clean, errands to run. All of that takes a lot of time and effort, too. You can re-prioritize and let some of it go but honestly a lot of it is necessary to be a good responsible parent!

I began talking to Eric about a process we learned about while undergoing fertility treatments. It is called "Snowflake Adoption." In Snowflake Adoption, you basically go through the adoption process of picking out a family for your frozen embryos. Infertile couples would then be able to undergo IVF with their adopted embryo. I felt a huge sense of responsibility to choose a loving, Christian family like ours for our embryos. Being infertile myself, I could see what a huge blessing it would be to another infertile couple.

I did not take this decision lightly by any means. I spent hours crying and praying about the it. We finally decided that we would continue to pray about it over the next few years. After Matthew started Kindergarten, we would decide one way or another. We did, however, go ahead and update our will. We needed to add Matthew's information. We also added a section pertaining to our embryos. If, by some tragic means, Eric and I were to both die, we gave custody of our embryos to my mom and my sister. They would then go through the Snowflake Adoption process and find a family for our embryos. When we finished explaining what we wanted to our lawyer he said, "Well this is certainly a new one for me!"

It probably sounds morbid that we even thought about that. I call it responsible. We were very proactive about doing everything that we could do to help create that life. That life that we know is a miracle. It was our responsibility to make sure that the embryos didn't just sit in cryopreservation indefinitely.

I watched my children grow up to be toddlers and preschoolers. Every day I would pray over them as well as my frozen embryos (our totsicles as we started to call them). Oh God, what would you have us do?

Chapter Six – A Change of Heart

August 2011

It had been a good, but very long, last few years. And finally the Greers had officially found their groove. I felt like I had the hang of raising three toddlers. We were moving and shaking. We went to the zoo, to the library, even McDonald's play land! I only had a meltdown every other day and that was usually because at least two Greer kids were having a meltdown, too.

I began to feel a bit restless about the next career steps God had planned for me. I added that to my daily prayer list. Every morning I prayed for direction and peace about what to do with our "totsicles". I also prayed for direction about my career. I knew I didn't want to go back to the corporate world. There was no halfway and I wasn't going back to working 50+ hour weeks. Did I need to go back to school? Was there something else I needed to do to prepare for the next step?

Ethan and Ella were a year away from starting Kindergarten and Matthew was ready to start preschool. I knew I wouldn't be content to stay at home while they were at school. However, I wasn't prepared to not be at home when they got home from school.

Eric's friend from work, Dennis, was married to a wonderful woman, Windy, who was the director of a fantastic preschool. She was always looking for new teachers that loved children. It sounded like a perfect match for me. I had thought about pursuing a degree in education before I went into business. And of course I loved children. Logistically it would be perfect. The kids could go to school at the preschool while I taught part-time.

I had met Dennis and Windy a few times before. They actually came to see me when I was in the hospital on bed rest with Ethan and Ella. They came at one of the few times that Eric left my side. They were so sweet and sat and talked to me even though I know it was an awkward situation! Unfortunately, they had also had their own battle with infertility. I had some phone conversations with Windy when she was going through treatments. It was also a time when Eric could really be a comfort to one of his friends about a very difficult topic for men to discuss.

The first school year was a blur but it was fantastic. I loved teaching. I loved the children. I loved the flexibility it gave me to still be there for everything with our kids. By the time Ethan and Ella attended their preschool graduation, I knew that this career was the path on which I needed to be.

Could I really do this??

During the months leading up to Ethan and Ella starting Kindergarten, I felt my heart start to shift. I had been adamant that I could not parent more than the children I already had and still be a good mom. As I began to think about two-thirds of the kids being in school five days a week, I felt a little hope.

As I watched Ethan and Ella become more independent, my hope grew. I finally got a chance to sit back sometimes and let them do for themselves.

My heart made the last turn to confidence when I babysat my friend, Whitney's, three boys. They were aged one, four, and six. I had six kids ranging in age from one to six at my house for a couple of hours. I am not going to lie. I was nervous before she dropped them off! But I was pleasantly surprised by how much easier it was to handle than I had anticipated. The older ones played well together. But the kicker was watching my sweet girl, Ella, help me with the baby. She was in love with Henry. Anything that she could do to help me, she was ready to do.

Full Heart Empty Womb

Now I was not so naive as to not realize that Henry was a novelty to her. I knew that the next day she might not want anything to do with him. And two hours of babysitting isn't the same as a lifetime with children. However, it dawned on me that I would have a little help. Even if it was just to grab a diaper for me. I never had that before! It wouldn't be like I had four or five infants. Three of them would have some independence.

I felt invigorated. Perhaps I could do this? And I realized that it wasn't just me – just Steph - anyway. Didn't I need a lot of prayer every day to get through my todays now? If God wanted me to have more than the three children He had already blessed me with, then He would help me through. That didn't mean that I wouldn't have bad days. I have bad days now. But He could help me get back up and start again.

I was excited and a little nervous to talk to Eric about my change of heart. It really was a 180 degree turn of attitude in just a few days. Would he just think I was over reacting to Ethan and Ella starting Kindergarten? Would he be worried about the financial strain of fertility treatments and more mouths to feed?

After we put the kids to bed, I took a deep breath and prepared to give the speech I had been rehearsing in my head all day. I spoke quickly outlining all of my thoughts, plans, and prayers so that I made sure he got my full picture before he rushed to judgment. After I finished my speech, I sat back and held my breath. I was completely surprised by his reaction. He smiled broadly and said, "That is what I wanted to do all along."

I was relieved and felt a little bit guilty. Would he really have let us give up our embryos for adoption when he wanted to keep them? Yes, he would, because he is a selfless man. He dried my tears during the years of failed cycles. He sat and watched me in the hospital for seventy-seven days. He took care of me in the last hours of my pregnancy with Ethan and Ella when I was in excruciating pain. He would not ever ask me to go through any of that again if I didn't want to. Even if it meant he would miss out on raising one of his children. How in the world did I get to be so blessed?

We decided that we needed to continue to pray about the decision for a while. We were so scared to make the wrong decision. And this decision was HUGE. It not only impacted us but our whole family. It even affected other families out there that we didn't even know.

What if I was just freaking out about my babies growing up? Was this feeling just an empty nest thing where I thought I was going to be lonely with them going to Kindergarten? I had been so sure that I was ready to place my embryos for adoption. Was I just being selfish and wanting to keep them for myself?

On the flip side, could I really go through fertility treatments again? I wasn't scared of the shots anymore. But the hormones and all the emotional baggage they entail! Could I handle that and still be a good mother to the three babies I already had?

The last time we went through fertility treatments we had two solid incomes and just Eric and I to support. Now, for the most part, we just had Eric's income. And we had three more mouths to feed and clothe. Fertility treatments are extremely expensive. We were comfortable, but we didn't have a lot of money to spare.

If I started to think about the possibility of having another high-risk pregnancy, I would nearly hyperventilate. I couldn't even think about being separated from my babies if I went into the hospital again. Of course I would follow doctor's orders, but it would be much harder when I have so many people that depend on me for *everything*! I spent hours worrying and crying in bed over what might or might not be.

I didn't have any issues with my second pregnancy, but I was only pregnant with one baby. If I did a FET with two embryos, then I *could* get pregnant with twins. Odds were that I would not get pregnant with twins, if at all. But honestly, I wanted to. I wanted *both of them*. The last time I did an embryo transfer, I did it with two embryos. One was Ethan and one was Ella. Which one of those would I be ok not having? *Neither.* They are both my sweet, precious babies. As much as the thought of it overwhelmed me, I wanted each and every one of my embryos.

So worst case scenario, what if I was hospitalized for a long time? I would miss out on precious time with my babies. They would miss their Mommy. Eric wouldn't be able to be my constant companion like he was last time. In fact, I probably would yell at him any time he came to the hospital because he needed to be at home with the kids when I couldn't. I ran every possible scenario over and over in my head each night. It was the same tear stained pillow as in 2005 but now it wasn't just our lives that would be affected. We had three children to think about, too.

Crystal Clear

We decided that it would be worth our time to meet with our Reproductive Endocrinologist, Dr. Whitworth, again to discuss how to proceed if we decided to keep our embryos. We learned that we had four embryos that were all graded well. She suggested that we thaw two at a time and possibly do two transfers.

This is one of the many times in our journey that our faith was literally our saving grace. I prayed. Eric prayed. I asked my parents and sister to pray for us, too. We even talked to our Sunday school teachers, Howard and Brenda, and asked them to pray for us. Over time, the right decision became crystal clear to Eric and me.

We made the decision to go forward with a Frozen Embryo Transfer (FET) of our four remaining embryos. We felt a peace about the decision once it was made. There was never a question of whether it was the right decision or not. Placing the embryos for adoption was no longer an option in my mind. It was a good option for another couple but not what God wanted for us.

Full Heart Empty Womb

We were excited about our decision but we weren't quite ready to begin the treatments. We thought we could wait a couple of years and save some money to help cover the costs of the procedures. Also, Matthew would then be in Kindergarten. Having a baby or babies at home would be a lot easier if the other three children were in school for at least part of the day.

When we shared our decision to proceed with the FET, we got a little push back from a few of our confidants. "Have you *even* thought about what would happen to the kids you have if you are put in the hospital again?" My answer: *constantly*. I had thought about little else than the "what ifs" for the past year. I cried myself to sleep many nights worrying about what could happen.

I remember one day being asked that very question - and what happened next. I was driving the kids home from Vacation Bible School. We were listening to the music that they were learning there. I was holding back my tears as I was praying for strength and God immediately answered that prayer. He reached out to me through the VBS music. A song came on and the kids started to sing, "If God is for me, who can be against me? Whatever happens I know that He is in control. If God is for me, who can be against me?" Immediately I felt a peace from the top of my head to the tips of my toes. God gave me a peace that He was right there with us every step of the way. People may not understand why we made the decision that we did, but God was there. God was for us and that was all that mattered. We were taking the path that He wanted us to and we were not alone. He was holding our shaking hands in His.

That didn't guarantee that it would be a smooth road. As difficult as my pregnancy with Ethan and Ella was, it had a wonderful outcome. I had two healthy children. That wasn't an absolute for the next time. I had to believe that if this was the path on which God was taking us, He would be there with us and help us overcome any obstacles than stood in our way.

My next step was to meet with my OBGYN, Dr. Blake, to discuss her opinion regarding the FET and a possible pregnancy. She was excited for us and our decision to pursue the FET. When I talked to her about waiting another couple of years, she shook her head. At the time, I was almost 35 years old. Even though my embryos were from a 28 year old, the body carrying those babies would be older. The older I was the harder the pregnancy would be on my body. My sales side emerged as I sat on the examining table and negotiated with her. "How about 18 months? A year? Oh, can we please at least wait until the beginning of the year?" We were planning our first trip to Disney World with the kids. I was afraid if we didn't go then, we would never be able to afford to go! She smiled and said that was fine.

I was nervous but I was excited. We were really doing this! How many more babies did God have in store for us? One? Two? FOUR? We spent the next several months saving, planning, and continuing to pray about our next steps.

Here We Go Again!

We had it all planned out. My cycles had been completely regular since I had Matthew. It was like he was my little Ctrl-Alt-Delete. He reset my body. Since my cycles were regular, we decided that I would do what is called a "natural IVF." A natural IVF is a method of IVF in which you do not use any drugs to control your cycle. You may have to have more ultrasounds so that in order to still time everything perfectly, the doctors can determine exactly at what point you are in your cycle. It would be so simple. I would do a natural IVF in January. If that didn't work, I would do the other natural IVF in February. That simple, right? When would I ever learn?

We decided to undergo a natural cycle for several reasons. First, we thought it was what was best for me, physically. I had so many drugs pumped into my body between my earlier fertility treatments and my pregnancy with Ethan and Ella. I was still feeling some lingering effects of those drugs. I never regretted taking them but if I could avoid it, then I certainly would. Also, the medications were incredibly expensive. If we could save thousands of dollars, you better believe we would!

Second, I did not want any of the hormonal effects that the drugs could produce. I was afraid that between the stress of the treatments and the mood swings, I would be even more emotional. The last thing I wanted to do was yell more at my kids or start to cry in front of them. Obviously they had no clue about what was going on. It wasn't an appropriate conversation to have with two Kindergarteners and a four-year-old!

The natural cycle was also my feeble attempt to let go and admit that I don't have control. We honestly believed that if God wanted me to get pregnant, then I would get pregnant. It didn't matter if I took a hundred shots that weren't entirely needed or not. Honestly, the fact that I had three babies at home made that acceptance much easier. At that point, I didn't have the burning desire to have a baby. I wasn't so desperate that I would do anything and everything just to have a baby anymore. I had the luxury to say that I would do what was necessary and leave the rest in God's hands.

Ringing in 2013

Our Christmas present to Ethan, Ella, and Matthew was to take them to Disney World over the New Year holiday. We were beyond excited. All of their friends had been. They never complained, but I knew they were dying to go. We were dying to take them! Going to Disney World was one of those experiences that I dreamed about enjoying with my children. We were so grateful that we were going to get a chance to do this trip before our life turned into complete chaos.

Full Heart Empty Womb

I was supposed to start my cycle at the end of our trip. Before we could proceed with the FET, I had to go to NFC for an ultrasound early in the cycle to make sure that I didn't have any cysts. My cycle had been like clockwork for the last couple of years, so I was sure that the timing would work. However, I started a little early so I missed the window for my ultrasound because we were out of town.

It was a letdown. We had been looking forward for the past few months to starting the process in January. I had even calculated that my due date would be in October. Another precious October baby!! I would now have to wait until February to begin the process. Again with the waiting game. Did waiting another month make that much of a difference? Not really. But it did feel like it. It ended up being a blessing in disguise, though. Eric had surgery at the beginning of February to repair a torn meniscus so I was able to give him my full attention before we started any treatments.

Round One...Ding Ding Ding!

So when I felt that first cramp in February, I was ecstatic! Here we go! My heart was literally racing as I called NFC to make my first appointment. I could not wait to get started. This was what we waited and prayed for and the time was *now*.

I remember sitting in the waiting room at NFC. I sat in my chair and looked around. I looked out the window and saw the beautiful Nashville skyline. How had I never noticed the amazing view from the office? I had been here countless times and never saw it. I looked back around at the people and knew why. There were various couples scattered all around the waiting room. Some were fiddling with their phones. Some were nervously leafing through magazines. All of them had their eyes cast downward and were broken and hurting. They were just trying to make it through the next ultrasound, the next blood test, the next step to hopefully having a baby. Immediately I was brought back to the emotions I felt so many years before. I prayed for their peace and their comfort.

I had my ultrasound and was declared cyst free and ready to go. I made an ultrasound appointment for a week or so later to try to determine when I was going to ovulate. They would need to be able to determine when I was going to ovulate so they could time the FET perfectly with my natural cycle.

While I waited a week for my next ultrasounds and blood work, I was simply energized. I was so excited and hopeful about the upcoming FET. After months of hoping and praying, I would know if I was pregnant in just a matter of weeks! I calculated due dates. I doodled different names on my grocery list. Amy Lynn, Charlotte, Noah, Nolan. I imagined what combination they would be of all of us. Would they have Ella's beautiful blue eyes? Matthew's grin with a dimple? Ethan's thick, wavy hair? I couldn't wait to see.

Some nights the excitement would turn to anxiety. Oh, what if I am separated from my babies and am put in the hospital? How can I make sure they are taken care of? Will we ask too much of our parents? They have already helped us so much! Where will the baby sleep? All our bedrooms are full. Can Ethan and Matthew share a room and not clobber each other? How are we going to afford another child?

I would stay up at night and plan. I would research room arrangements so that the boys would be happy and black eye free in their tighter quarters. I resolved to go back to being the best bargain shopper in town. I decided I would work more days at the preschool. Anything I could do to take some of the financial burden off Eric's shoulders. If we had to, we would move to a more affordable area. I would think and plan until my anxiety passed. Ideally I would fall back asleep before it was time to get up and start the day. If not, I poured myself a big Diet Coke to chug as I started making breakfasts, lunches, and snacks for three kids. Sometimes I remembered to feed myself, too.

Full Heart Empty Womb

I returned for an ultrasound on cycle day 11. They were examining my follicles to try to determine when I was going to ovulate. They also looked at the lining of my uterus to make sure it was thickening as it should for an ideal cycle. Before my ultrasound they always took some blood to check my hormone levels. I was encouraged by my ultrasound results. My lining was thick and looked to be right where it needed to be. I was still not quite ready to ovulate so I made another appointment to come back in a couple of days to check on the growth of my follicles. These results were what I expected to hear so I was excited. Everything seemed to be on course for our FET in the next week. On the way home I called my mom to give her a heads up so that she could help with the kids during the transfer.

I almost forgot to call my voicemail box later that afternoon to check on my blood work. Everything looked good so I didn't think about it. I didn't call until the office closed. I picked up the voicemail from my IVF nurse, Jordan, which told me that my estrogen level was quite low. It was unusual for my estrogen to be low with a thick lining. Low estrogen would normally cause a thin endometrial lining. Since the picture wasn't quite lining up, she wanted Dr. Whitworth to do the ultrasound scan herself.

I tried to not let it get to me, but I couldn't help it. What was wrong with me? I did what they always tell you not to do and googled, "Low Estrogen". I found all kinds of good news about PCOS, possible menopause, eating disorders, (which was laughable) and even one article hinted at cancer which immediately made me freak out. What in the world else is wrong with me? What if the whole reason I was going through this process was to find out there was something else far worse wrong with me? I immediately started thinking about the worst-case scenarios.

I called my best friend, Jodi, crying. She asked me if Eric was going with me to my next appointment. I said that I didn't want to bother him. There would be a lot of appointments and he couldn't miss work. Then she did what every best friend would do. She went behind my back and told Eric that he needed to go to the ultrasound with me.

Full Heart Empty Womb

I was glad she did. I was freaking out inside. I had so many "what ifs" going through my head. I knew some of the thoughts I was having were irrational, but I couldn't stop my mind from racing. I had my three kids to think about. It wasn't just Eric and me anymore. And how come I couldn't even be considered normal in the infertility world?

Eric came with me to the appointment and kept me sane. He made little comments in his sarcastic way and made me laugh. We aren't a handholding couple, but he held my hand in the waiting room as we stared at the double doors waiting for my name to be called. He made small talk with the nurses as we walked back and made them laugh. He was completely at ease and his calm presence made the knot in my stomach loosen. Here we were again eight years later in an ultrasound room together. I still made Eric turn around when I disrobed from the waist down until I was covered in my paper blanket. Now we stared at the ultrasound machine and weren't horrified. We were curious. What are you going to tell us is wrong now?

Dr. Whitworth came in to do our scan. She explained that she liked to do the scan if the ultrasounds and blood work had conflicting information. I appreciated having her there so I could get her opinion immediately. She was able to tell fairly quickly what our issue was. A portion of the top of my endometrial lining was irregular and had fluid present so it indicated there might be an endometrial polyp. Fortunately she was able to test further immediately. She performed a hydro sonogram, which appeared to be normal, so we could rule out the endometrial polyp. In a hydro sonogram, the doctor injects a saline solution into the uterus to get a better look at the uterus and lining. We decided that because there was fluid present and my follicles weren't developing as well as they should, we would cancel the cycle. We also decided that with the next cycle we would still do a natural cycle but we would add Femara (a FSH) to help the follicles develop better.

It was a letdown for sure. I cried a few tears but put on my happy face. I chastised myself for thinking that it would be this easy. We had waited this long; what was one more month? Seriously? It is forever.

The next few weeks lasted forever! I felt like all I was doing was waiting and wishing. I was literally wishing my life away.

Round Two.....Ding! Ding! Ding!

Again we began. We were excited at first. I was excited when I got my drugs! Here we go!! I was so proud of myself that I even gave myself my own shots! I definitely had to give myself a pep talk but I did it. I locked myself in my bathroom early in the mornings so that I didn't risk any of the kids walking in and seeing it. I hid all my supplies up high in my bathroom cabinet behind a bunch of towels.

When I went in for my lining check, I felt positive. I was sure that the addition of the Femara had been what I needed. It would give my follicles the needed boost to mature and my lining would be thick and smooth like it needed to be. Wrong. The follicles were better but I still had fluid in my lining. They asked me to come back the next day for a scan with Dr. Whitworth again so she could see for herself.

Dr. Whitworth did my scan and saw there was still fluid in my uterus. Cycle cancelled again. She was very caring and could tell that I was very disappointed. I tried to smile through my tears as we talked through our next steps. Apparently doing a natural IVF cycle was not going to work for me. We would try it again the next cycle but we would do the full IVF cocktail. I would start with the suppression drugs (my personal fav) the next cycle. The following cycle I would start the FSH drugs. So that meant it would be TWO MONTHS before I had the chance to do my first FET. That is *five* months after I thought I would be able to have my first one.

Oh, I was exhausted. It was mentally draining to get my hopes up and dashed over and over. It was hard to try to get everything lined up for childcare just in case. I had plans for different days of the week between my mom and Sarah. Both were more than willing to help but

I hated to have them put their lives on hold, too. Then of course I had to keep my boss, Windy, in the loop so she knew when I would need off work. Fortunately she was very supportive and gave me whatever time I needed.

I was also physically exhausted. The lack of sleep and stress on my body was taking its toll on me. I was running a hundred miles an hour during the day trying to take care of the kids. I didn't want what I was going through to take away anything from them. I worked my butt off until I laid them down to bed and then I crashed myself.

That was generally when the tears came. I was too tired to hold them back. And I finally didn't have to hide them from anyone. I cried about why I couldn't be normal. Why couldn't I even be normal enough to do IVF for goodness sake? I thought it was going to be so simple. Why did everything have to be so hard? I had felt so good about doing a natural IVF. I thought it was a mature, responsible decision. We weren't trying to take control of the situation this time. Well look where that got us. Drugs and needles galore. Just FIVE months later.

Time Out

So I did what every sane woman does when she needs a good distraction. I redecorated. We had moved into a fixer upper a couple of years before. We moved to a different part of town that had the best schools. It was much pricier than where we first lived, so we got a house that we loved but that needed a lot of love. We tackled a couple of big projects in the beginning but had to put the rest on hold to pay for the infertility treatments.

Our playroom was decorated pretty much like it was Eric's playroom. Everything was University of Tennessee. Orange and white were everywhere. Now, I love the VOLS, but I was ready to reclaim the largest room in our house. Since we were in the midst of infertility treatments, my budget wasn't very big. I channeled my inner "Trading Spaces" designer and worked with what I had. I rearranged furniture. I painted walls. I sprung for a few new throw pillows. In the end, my playroom was transformed from Neyland Stadium to my own little beach oasis. It seems silly, but it gave me a project. Something else to focus on besides the wasted time and the upcoming FET.

Round Three…Ding!! Ding!! Ding!!

By the time I started Lupron, the suppression drug, my emotions were very close to the surface. I remember sitting in Sunday school and repeatedly blinking back the tears. My teacher, Howard, had asked if anyone had anything big going on that week. It was an innocent enough question. Inside I was crying because I started my Lupron injections that week. I couldn't even keep control of my tears. Thankfully it was allergy season so I could blame it on that. My friend, Ashley, knew better though. She sent me a text as soon as we left church encouraging me.

I gave myself all of the Lupron injections since they were subcutaneous injections. However, they switched my FSH to a stronger drug to ensure my lining would thicken as we needed it to. This drug was an intramuscular shot. My progesterone was an IM shot too. There were some days when I had two IM shots in my hip. Those days and the ones following were pretty tough because I couldn't alternate and give a side a break. My backside was incredibly sore and looked like I had been beaten from all the bruising!

The effects of the shots were just as I remembered from the first go around. I had horrible hot flashes that kept me up at night. I didn't need any help in that department. My mind was already racing with "what ifs" all night long. I remember sitting at one of Matthew's baseball games and thinking, "I am literally going to drop right now." I had worked all day in a very active job. I went straight to pick up the kids and did homework with Ethan and Ella immediately when we got home. I got everyone to eat a quick dinner before we all left for the ballpark. I was beyond exhausted. I finally got the true meaning of the expression "running on empty."

It was all worth it when we finally got the green light and a transfer date. It was in the middle of May. It was a crazy time with the end of school for the kids and me, but it worked out for the best. My transfer was on the day of Matthew's end of year class party. Fortunately I was able to drop him off at his party and my mom could pick him up. Since school was ending I wouldn't have to go back to work. I didn't have to worry about any explanations for time off or lifting restrictions at work so that took a lot of stress off of me. The big kids would still be in school for a little while so I could take it easy post-transfer.

Eric and I were just giddy the day of the transfer. We were finally here! After all this time, setbacks, and prayer we were finally to the day of transfer. We giggled as Eric got dressed in his scrubs to come back for the transfer with me. He even posed for a picture for me.

I had been separated from my little totsicles for over seven years now. The embryologist came into our room with a picture and report on our embryos. They had thawed and looked good! He had a picture for us to keep. We smiled at our little bubble pictures. "Who are you?" I thought. "Are you Amy Lynn? Noah? Or maybe two girls or two boys!!" I was excited to be reunited with them soon. I held the picture of my totsicles to my chest, whispered a prayer, and actually fell asleep for a few minutes before the transfer. I was at such peace with the whole situation. I knew this was in God's hands.

The transfer went smoothly. I was so nervous about the time following the transfer. I remembered how uncomfortable I had been last time with having such a full bladder. This time I wasn't the least bit uncomfortable and actually slept most of the time! It was a nice surprise.

Full Heart Empty Womb

On the way home, Eric picked up my favorite meal just like he had so many years before. He got me set up in my bed with a TV tray, remotes, my Kindle, and my iPhone so I could relax for the rest of the day. I ate my big ole salad, rubbed my belly, and told my babies that I would take good care of them. They just had to stick around. I drifted off to sleep with my hands on my belly where they essentially stayed the next two weeks.

When the kids got home they all climbed in bed with me. We told them that I had hurt my back so I had to take it easy a couple of days. I didn't have two days of bed rest this time. The restrictions had gotten a little lighter since my first time with IVF. I was going to stay on bed rest that day. The next several days I would take it easy as much as I could. They didn't say that I had to, I just wanted to. Last time that is what I did and I got pregnant, so I didn't want to stray too far from that!

That being said, taking it easy with three small kids is difficult. Just to get three kids fed and out the door to school is more activity than a lot of people see in a day! I did the best that I could though. As soon as I got Ethan and Ella off to school, I came home and rested on the couch with Matthew. He was in heaven because he pretty much got a free pass to watch TV and read books with me all day long. The lifting restrictions were the hardest for me. Even though Matthew was four years old, I still picked him up a lot. I couldn't help it. When he was tired, sometimes it was just easier to pick him up. And he gave the best hugs in the world. They were full body hugs where he would jump up and wrap his legs and arms around me and squeeze with all his might. They were his Spider Monkey hugs. I was still getting my Spider Monkey hugs, but I was just sitting on the couch.

After a few days, I started to resume a more normal schedule although I still followed the lifting restrictions. Once, I was in the grocery store with Matthew and I had a little panic attack. Matthew stood next to the cart with his arms outstretched to me ready to get in the cart. I couldn't help him get in the cart because I couldn't lift him. I looked back at my extremely long list and back at him. I hadn't been to the grocery store for a real trip since before the transfer. When it was just Eric and me, we could live on takeout. With the kids we had to make sure we had good nutritious meals and snacks each day. Fortunately Matthew was thrilled to walk around the grocery store like a big boy. And I only found a few things that he had thrown in the cart when I wasn't looking!

I also started to feel different. My breasts were extremely sensitive. I couldn't even sleep on my stomach because they hurt too much. Of course that was tricky because my bottom was sore from all the injections. I ended up sleeping on my side until I rolled over and woke up in pain. I didn't care though because sore boobies meant I could be pregnant!! The next day I would feel a cramp in my belly and freak out thinking I was about to start. I would chastise myself for getting too excited. I knew the progesterone shots could cause side effects that mimic pregnancy symptoms! It really was quite cruel.

By the time I went in for my beta test on Memorial Day, I was convinced I was pregnant. My breasts were still very sore and I was very tired. I just knew those were signs I was pregnant. I went to have my blood drawn and then I came back to the house to get Ella. I took her to a nail salon so that we could have our nails done and pass the time. Eric had the boys at home. They were blowing up our big inflatable pool to have a big first day of summer bash in the backyard. By the time Ella and I got home it was about time to call and get my results.

We quickly prepared the kids their lunch and ran back to our bedroom to make the call into our voicemail box. We huddled up next to each other on our bed and dialed the number and held our breath. We smiled and giggled as I fumbled over the numbers through the voicemail prompts. My fingers were shaking with excitement. When we heard that I had a message, we shrieked. We would know for sure any second! My hands grasped my belly, my *babies*.

Our hearts sank when the nurse came on the line and said that my beta number was two and that it had to be at least 50 for it to be considered

Full Heart Empty Womb

positive. I was nowhere near pregnant. My body wasn't trying to tell me that I was pregnant. It was those *stupid, stupid* drugs. My hands dropped from my empty womb. I cried. I sobbed. I wailed. Eric wrapped me in his arms and rubbed my back. I heard a soft cry from him. He told me he really thought I was pregnant too.

We took a deep breath. As badly as we were hurting, there were three precious kids that were waiting to have the time of their lives once they finished their mac and cheese. Eric said he would get them outside playing while I pulled myself together and called my parents.

My hands were shaking as I dialed my parents but it wasn't from excitement this time. I imagined my mom sitting expectantly by the phone all morning. I am sure she jumped in anticipation every time the phone rang. Being a planner like me, I am sure she had already designed the quilt she was going to make her new grandbaby or grandbabies! When she answered the phone with an excited, "Hello!" I knew she thought I was pregnant, too. It only took a sob from me to correct that notion. I honestly don't remember our conversation. I was in a haze of sadness, but I know it did give me the strength to stop the tears.

Five minutes later I was walking outside to pretend like everything was ok. That was all the time I got to say goodbye to the babies I had been so sure I was carrying. I had other babies that were ready for a backyard bash for whom I had to be strong. Matthew ran up to me and gave me a Spider Monkey hug. He quickly apologized because he was afraid he hurt my back. I pulled him up close and told him that my back was all better. I let a single tear fall for the baby brother or sister that he would not have.

Eric had the pool blown up and full of freezing cold water from the hose. The kids didn't care. They laughed and splashed like they were at the most grand pool in the world. He had a couple of chairs set up for us and had a cold beer for me in my favorite coozie. I sat back and let the warm May sun wash over my face. We were sitting close enough to watch the kids but far enough that we could talk without them hearing. I asked him to take care of letting everyone else know. He would call his family and send an email to Howard and Brenda, our Sunday school teachers. I was just talked out. I couldn't tell the story anymore. I couldn't listen to the well intentioned words or condolences. I couldn't put on the happy face and say all the "Christian" things I was supposed to say.

I watched the kids play in the pool and on the rope swing and my mind started to process what happened. I was sad because those were two of our babies that we would never know. Babies that I loved and prayed for daily. I was so grateful to be able to spend the day with the three babies that I did have. I never lost sight of the blessings they were, but I still mourned the babies I thought I would have.

My mind continued to tick as I sat in my lawn chair. "This isn't over yet". I still have two more embryos. Maybe this is for the best? I could handle raising four or five children better than seven! Oh, I feel horrible that I even just thought that! Of course I would rather be pregnant right now! But since I am not, I don't have to worry about going through fertility treatments again in a couple of years with the last two embryos! Gosh! I can't believe I thought that. Of course I would do that if it meant I could have all my babies." I sat there and mentally beat myself up for having the most natural thoughts.

At the end of the day after we put three very tired, happy kids to bed, I let the tears fall that I had kept bottled up for the last ten hours. I cried because I wanted those babies. Then I cried because I felt guilty because I had three awesome kids. How could I be sad? But it just didn't change the fact that I saw each of those embryos as my baby and now I would never get to hold them and love them. Eric held me as I cried until I had no tears.

When I ran out of tears, I gained determination. We were fortunate. This was not the end of the road for us. We decided that we would jump right back on the horse and immediately do another FET. If I started Lupron in June, then I could do my FET in July before we started school again. It would be so much simpler for us to plan. I wouldn't have to miss work. The kids could just go see their Nana and Papa or Mimi and PaPa during the transfer and be none the wiser about what was going on with me. We had a plan so I felt better.

I never anticipated how hard it would be to go through fertility treatments while already raising kids. I remembered that on my online support website, there was a section called "Secondary Infertility" that was separate from everyone else. I am embarrassed to admit my lack of sympathy for them at the time. I remember thinking, "Yes, but at least you have a child." That is very true. The comfort that my children brought me was immeasurable. I was not at the point of desperation to have a child like I was the first time.

However, having children who depend on you and at the same time going through the stress of infertility is extremely hard. You have to have your game face on all the time. You can't break down into tears when the hormones and emotions overtake you. They are children. They don't need my baggage. And you are not just juggling your schedule with doctor appointments, you are juggling theirs, too. Don't even get me started on the Mommy Guilt! As much pressure as you put on yourself to get pregnant – you put that much and more to be the best parent possible. Handling the stress of cycling while still giving 110% to your kids is grueling. I never felt like there was enough of me. I am not sure why we as a society feel like we need to put a person's emotional pain on a scale. Some people's pain may be more, some may be less. Pain is pain.

Going Down the Tubes

I got a call from Dr. Whitworth later that week. She wanted me to have a hysterosalpingogram (HSG) to see if there was anything else going on that may have contributed to my failed FET. Like many other tests, I had to wait for a certain cycle day to schedule it. We were getting closer and closer to our family vacation and I still was not able to schedule it. It was so stressful. If I didn't start soon, we would either have to cancel our vacation or wait to do the test another month. I couldn't cancel the vacation! We needed it too much. Our family needed a break to just be together and enjoy each other. Waiting another month was not good either. If we waited another month, that would put my transfer during the middle of school. That would add a lot of complications to the situation. Oh, the stress of the waiting and scheduling! I felt like this was my life!

Fortunately, I started and was able to do the test two days before we left on vacation. They did the test at a surgery center and the results were sent to Dr. Whitworth to read. She would call me in a few days to discuss. Unfortunately, that also meant that the test results were weighing heavily on me while we were away. We had a great vacation, although my iPhone was glued to my hand. Every time my phone rang I jumped and looked at the caller ID.

One day Ethan came up to me and asked me to go on a walk with him on the beach. Of course there was nothing I wanted to do more. I stood up with my iPhone, looked down at it then threw it back on my chair. He deserved 100% of my attention. We walked up and down the beach. We talked about everything and about absolutely nothing hand in hand. It was a sweet time.

We got back from our walk and he went back to digging in the sand while I went back to my chair by the water. I moved my iPhone to sit down and saw "1 missed call and Voice Mail" on the screen. Well crap. Isn't that just my luck? I motioned to Eric and started running towards the stairs to our room where we had better cell reception. I repeatedly tried to dial the number without success as I sprinted toward our room. When I finally was able to pick up the message, it was Dr. Whitworth. Between my nerves and the message cutting out, I got a few pieces of the puzzle: "pockets of fluid in my uterus - - surgery- - tubes may need to be removed." WHAT??!! My mind was so jumbled. I didn't understand. My tubes were tied after I had Matthew! How could they be the problem? Surgery! No. No. No!! I quickly called the office and left what I was sure was a crazy message for my IVF nurse, Jordan. I

105

saw that it was the time the office was closing so I knew I wouldn't hear back until the next day.

That night was long. It wasn't until after we put the kids to bed that we could sit and talk about things. I had kept things bottled up, and they were simmering all day ready to burst. I wished I had been able to talk to Dr. Whitworth so I could understand what was going on. But that wasn't going to stop me from trying to figure it out on my own until I talked to her!

We sat out on our patio and had what was probably the biggest argument of our marriage. I knew she had mentioned that I might need to have my fallopian tubes removed. I was conflicted. We started this process trying to be as minimally invasive as possible. Now we were talking about voluntarily removing part of my body? But if there was something wrong that I could fix, didn't I have the responsibility to the embryos to give them every chance they had to implant? If I didn't have the tubes removed and I knew that decreased their chances to implant, wouldn't that be just like throwing them away? Didn't I owe them the best chance possible?

Eric was adamant that I had put my body through enough. He didn't want me to hurt any more than I already had. He was worried about not only the surgery itself, but the long term repercussions of removing part of my female reproductive organs. I already had what I believed where side effects from all of the drugs I had been on from the preterm labor. What if I were to go straight into menopause at such an early age? He was very concerned about how it would affect my quality of life long term. I said that I couldn't be selfish like that. We went back and forth with a lot of tears. I felt like he was fighting for me and I was fighting for the babies. Finally we decided that we just needed to go in and talk to Dr. Whitworth as soon as we got back and get all the information. This decision we should have reached from the beginning, but it is hard to just sit on a big piece of information like that.

The next day we went to lunch before taking the kids on a pirate cruise. Argh! My phone rang. It was Jordan returning my call. She quickly explained to me what the issue was so I understood. Because of where my fallopian tubes had been tied, there was an enzyme that was leaking back into my uterus. That was making pockets of fluid in my uterine lining, which would make it very difficult for an embryo to implant. We made an appointment for first thing the following Monday to discuss the test results more thoroughly and possible treatment options.

Eric and I decided to put the issue to rest until after we had all the facts from Dr. Whitworth. I wish I had had the sense to do that from the beginning. I was always trying to figure things out and make a plan. It was one of the most difficult things about infertility for me. I couldn't plan for anything. We decided to go back to what worked for us. We would pray about the situation and let God give us the guidance on which direction to go. By the time we got to our meeting on Monday morning we felt at peace.

Dr. Whitworth showed us the pictures from the HSG and explained exactly what the issue was. Usually when a patient gets her tubes tied, it is solely as a means of birth control. Regardless of whether the tubes are tied right up next to the uterus or a little further back, the job is done. However, it has already been established that Stephanie Greer is not just anyone. I needed my tubes tied for two reasons: avoid a natural pregnancy (even though that would truly be a miracle like with Matthew) and interfering with my future fertility treatments. Since my tubes had been tied a bit back from my uterus it was allowing an enzyme to leak back into my uterus thus making my lining uneven with pockets of fluid.

We talked about possible treatment options. Could we just untie them? Unfortunately, no. It wasn't as simple as that. Could we cut out the tie, attach them back together so that I could keep my fallopian tubes? No again. The fallopian tubes are not the same diameter all around so they wouldn't line up. That scenario could open us up to a whole host of possible complications. The best option was to just have them removed. Dr. Whitworth assured us that the fallopian tubes had nothing to do with any of my female hormones. It would not cause early menopause or anything of that nature.

She also explained that it could be done through a laparoscopic surgery on an outpatient basis. I had already had a "lap" before my first round of fertility treatments and remembered it not being a big deal. We felt much better about the situation. It was not going to harm me long term and would provide us a solution to fix the lining issue that had plagued us. I had to wait until I started a new cycle so that they could time the surgery well before ovulation.

So here we were waiting again. We waited for test results. Now we were waiting for my next cycle. Then we would wait for my surgery. Then summer would be over. I felt like I was wishing and waiting my life away. Of course I made the most of the time that I had. I never wanted what I was going through to take anything away from the kids. If anything, that guilt drove me to overdo it. I was constantly planning something for the kids so that they could have the best summer possible. Remember that Mommy Guilt I mentioned?

Week after week passed. Of course since my cycle was always on schedule, I was completely off schedule now when I least needed to be. After I was a week late, I emailed Jordan. Dr. Whitworth and I had tentatively planned on doing the surgery the next week. I hadn't even started yet! I was hoping I could do it then because it would have worked perfectly. It was the one week all summer when I had the kids in a day camp. They could be having fun and learning while I was having my surgery. I wouldn't have to worry about finding someone to watch them. I could be back home and in bed "sick" so they wouldn't even know what happened. Jordan prescribed me some Prometrium to help induce my cycle. I thought it was ironic that the same drug that I took to help me stay pregnant was the drug that I was going to take to help me start my period…so I could get my fallopian tubes removed…so I could have a shot at getting pregnant…via fertility treatments. What? Some people have sex to get pregnant??

Full Heart Empty Womb

When you take Prometrium to start your cycle, you can take it one day and then start or you could take it ten days and start after that. Where do you think I landed? Ten days. I was three full weeks late this cycle. Yes, now we had completely missed the day camp window and now I was just worried about getting my surgery scheduled before my kids started back to school.

I finally was able to get it scheduled a couple of days before our 11th anniversary and one week before Ethan and Ella started 1st grade. It wasn't ideal, but our parents were there to help us through. The kids were thrilled because they got to live up their last weekend before school started getting spoiled by their grandparents!

The day before the surgery, I wanted to get in my last bit of fun with them. I knew I wasn't going to be up to a lot of big outings after it. We met my friend, Devon, and her kids and played at the park. We ended it with lunch at Chik-Fil-A. I couldn't have asked for a better last meal than a Southern Fried Chicken Sandwich!

I took the kids off to have their fun. Then I sat down and started with my fun – drinking the magnesium citrate. I had learned a thing or two since the last time I did it. Last time it hit me at about two a.m. and I was up for the rest of the night. I was determined to speed up the process this time. I chugged water too. I got on my elliptical machine and had a Netflix marathon as I willed my bowels to get moving a little quicker. Eric worked late that night since he would be taking the next day off. He got home around ten and I was sweaty and had walked a gazillion miles on my elliptical. He looked at me like I was completely crazy!

My plan kind of worked. My surgery wasn't until noon, so I was able to get a little bit of sleep. We went in to the surgery center excited. One more step closer! Get these tubes outta me so we can move on to our FET!

I remember slowly coming out of the anesthesia after the surgery. My throat was scratchy and my belly was sore. Eric was there holding my hand. Dr. Whitworth was able to remove my fallopian tubes with no issue. She did see that I had an enormous amount of scar tissue from my two previous C-sections. That is not at all uncommon for C-sections. The amount that I had was more than most though. It was so much that my uterus was actually attached to my bladder. She spent time trying to remove some, but in the end it was too thick and viscous to cut through.

Eric got me home and in bed. I was so tired that I slept most of the day. When I woke I was very sore. We stayed on top of my pain meds because I was so uncomfortable. I couldn't even get out of bed by myself for the first couple of days. I took Motrin as soon as I could and then stared at the clock until it was time to take another pill. I was caught off guard by how much pain I was in. I didn't remember it being anywhere near this bad with the last lap that I had.

The last surgery I had I only took a long weekend off from work and was ready to go back to work on Monday. Granted going back to work for me was sitting in my home office at my laptop. I had anticipated the same so I had the kids come back Sunday night. I was thrilled to see them. Nothing made me happier than to see my babies' faces. I was nervous though about taking care of them on my own Monday.

Before Eric left for work he made sure the kids were fed. I loaded up on my Motrin and got ready to face the day. I wasn't comfortable taking a pain pill with him gone. They made me too groggy. We took it easy and watched some cartoons. Because my stomach was so sore, they couldn't even sit on my lap. They thought it was because I hurt my back again. After we watched a little TV, I started to feel guilty. They only had a few days left of summer. I couldn't make them sit in front of the TV! So I got out a lawn chair and sat in my jammies out on the driveway while they played. I was so swollen from the surgery that I couldn't even wear any of my clothes. I was so sore the idea of a waistband on my incision made me cringe.

My sweet friend, Whitney, came to my rescue. She brought me some of her old maternity clothes with a nice soft stretchy waistband that I could wear as I healed. Added to that, she brought me a big old Sonic Diet Coke since I told her how tired I was! I appreciated her taking the time to take care of me. And I needed clothes because I was going to have to leave the house in a couple of days for the kids' back to school ice cream social.

The ice cream social was a fun time for Ethan and Ella to see their friends and also find out who their teacher was going to be that year. They had been looking forward to it for weeks. I knew that I couldn't handle trying to wrangle Matthew and give Ethan and Ella the attention they deserved. I had my mom come over to play with Matthew. And I am so glad I did.

I was still in a considerable amount of pain. My pain was just as great five days post op as it was the day of surgery. I had to park far away from the school because there were so many people there. The kids ran ahead me up the hill to the school. It wasn't a steep hill by any means, but it felt like I was climbing a mountain. I moved slowly while clutching my right side where the pain was the greatest. I called to them to wait for me at the top of the hill. By the time I got to the top of the hill, I was holding back tears. Not only was this the longest distance I had walked in almost a week, but I was in the most pain I had been in to date. I blinked back the tears and put on my game face for the kids. I stood in a crowded, hot cafeteria as the kids chatted with their friends and ate their sweet treats. I felt sweat drip down my legs and I glanced down to make sure it wasn't blood. I was in so much pain that I was sure that I had popped a stitch or something. I smiled. I made small talk with moms. I glanced at my watch to see if we had been there long enough.

Once we were in the car, I let the tears fall as Ethan and Ella talked eagerly in the back on the way home. They were so excited about being "Graders"! No more Kindergarteners. When we walked into the house, my mom knew immediately how much pain I was in. I headed straight to the freezer to get my ice pack and went to my healing station. I turned my heating pad on high and sat back on it in my recliner. I wrapped my icepack on my right side that was throbbing. It was dinnertime and my mom graciously offered to stay and get the kids fed. I cried and protested feebly. She took the kids and had them fed, bathed, and ready for bed by the time Eric got home. I was so grateful. As soon as Eric got home, I took a pain pill and went immediately to bed.

On the first day of school I made Ethan and Ella a big breakfast like I always do. We walked them into school with huge smiles on their faces. I collapsed back in my recliner with my heating pad and ice pack when we got home. I had gotten over my TV guilt. Matthew and I watched Disney Jr. all the way up until we went to go pick them up from school. The first day was a half-day, so I wanted to take the kids out to lunch for a treat. We rarely eat out so they really think it is special when we do.

About half way through our meal I was almost doubled over in pain. I started to consider if I needed to just get Eric to meet me at the ER. I knew this couldn't be right. Should I really be in this much pain a week after the surgery? Eric encouraged me to call Jordan. She returned my phone call immediately. She told me that I could be in pain for 10 to 14 days. I really needed to take it easy and take the pain pills. I had stopped taking them too early and that was why I was in so much pain. Because she had done so much maneuvering to get at the extra scar tissue, I was bruised pretty badly. That was why it hurt so badly on the right side. The surgical tools were inserted through this incision on my right side. Eric came home early so I could take my pain pills and get in bed. After a weekend of really taking it easy, I was feeling better. Not great, but I could function.

I simply didn't give myself enough time to heal. I should have spoken up at the beginning of the week when I was struggling. I thought that surely it was going to get better. I am sure that Sarah or my mom would have dropped everything to come and help us. But it was my silly pride that got in the way. I was the Mommy and I had to be the one to do this and that for my babies. I couldn't let my situation get in the way of being the Mommy I was supposed to be. In reality that is exactly what I did. My stubbornness to do it all on my own landed me sick in bed and in an extreme amount of pain.

Game Plan

I came to Eric with an idea that had been milling around in my head the last few days. I wanted to see if Dr. Whitworth would be willing to let us try a natural FET with no drugs this time. Since I had my fallopian tubes removed, that should have also removed my main issue with the fluid in the lining. If I could do a natural FET, that would eliminate at least some of the physical, emotional, and financial pain of it. I ended my explanation to Eric with, "I am not trying to be lazy. I will do all the shots if I need to." It is insane that I actually had guilt about even exploring if there was a possibility that I didn't have to take all the shots. We decided to pray about it and see what Dr. Whitworth had to say.

By the time I had my two week checkup with Dr. Whitworth I felt a ton better. She explained to me that the scar tissue was why I was sorer than I expected to be. She also said that the scar tissue would not be an issue for me unless I had another C-section. If I were to get pregnant then it would be very important that the doctors be aware of the extra scar tissue before delivery. "Ah ha!" I thought. That is why the surgery was so much more difficult! It was going to save me more pain down the road when I got pregnant! It was like a sign to me.

When we talked to Dr. Whitworth about the idea to try another natural IVF, she was supportive of our idea. It would involve more blood work and ultrasounds so that they could determine where I was in my cycle and time the transfer accordingly. Granted, statistically speaking we had a slightly better chance of getting pregnant if I were to take all of the drugs. I was at a point where I was completely at peace with that. My faith that God was in control of this process was stronger than any percentage point. He had given me a peace about pursuing the last FET with no drugs.

Dr. Whitworth also told us that we would have to wait eight weeks post op to do another FET in order to let the internal stitches heal. I should have realized that I couldn't hop right into another transfer after the surgery but I didn't. I fully anticipated that I would get to do one in September.

It turned out to be a very good thing that we weren't able to do another FET for another month. Since Matthew was born, Eric had been dealing with diverticulitis. It started with an episode here and there and steadily got worse. They would last for a couple of weeks and he was in a great deal of pain. We looked into surgery, but it didn't seem right early on. It was a very invasive surgery with a lengthy hospital stay and recovery. He could take medicine for it, but the side effects from it were just as bad as the diverticulitis. He had a particularly bad attack that September. Although he was in an excruciating amount of pain, he would never miss work. He would call me some nights and say that he would be later because he couldn't drive home. It was horrible.

We decided that it had gotten bad enough that we had to explore the surgery again. We met with the surgeon and got him scheduled for a colon resection in mid-November. That was as soon as he could have it done because his colon had to have some time to heal after the diverticulitis attack he had just suffered.

We contemplated putting off the FET that we had planned for October. In the end we decided that we had to just proceed. I am quite sure that our family thought we were crazy. But Eric and I were on the same page. We had let this rule our lives for long enough. If we waited then we would have to wait until at least January. And there is no "taking time off" when you are dealing with infertility. It is always right there in your mind. I think that is something that you don't understand unless you have lived through it. I didn't want it to be weighing me down over the holidays. I wanted to be able to focus on my family without distraction.

This is IT!!

When I started my cycle I had the same surge of excitement that I got every time we began a treatment. After all this *waiting* and praying this is it! We are finally moving forward! I mentally figured when my transfer would most likely be. I made tentative arrangements for the kids with my mom and Sarah. I put the transfer date in a due date calculator and saw I would have a June baby. Just like me!

I didn't go into the office until cycle day eleven, so it felt a little slow-going at first. Boy did we make up for it! I had blood work and an ultrasound to see how close I was to ovulation. Since I wasn't using any drugs they had already prepared me that I may need to come in more than once to be able to pinpoint when my body was going to naturally ovulate. When the ultrasound tech asked me if this was my first day, I knew it was a bad sign. My endometrium was basically non-existent and there was fluid present. Fluid?? I felt like I was going to lose it! I had a very painful surgery not long ago to correct my fluid problem! They asked me to come back on Monday to see if there was any improvement. I was devastated. I was sure that my cycle was going to be canceled. I was angry because I could still see my healing incisions on my belly and I thought, "Why did I go through all that pain for nothing?"

It was a long, long weekend. Again I was waiting. I didn't even have a lot of hope. In my mind I was just waiting to get canceled on Monday. When I went in on Monday, there was a slight improvement. My follicle had grown a little bit. My endometrium was still thin but the fluid had gotten smaller. We were cautiously optimistic and they had me come back in on Tuesday.

Tuesdays are a day that I teach so I had to go in late to work. Eric took Matthew into school while I was getting my ultrasound. Again I was so grateful that Windy was so understanding about our situation. Eric still had to answer some questions about where I was when he brought Matthew in. It was so hard to be going through such a huge situation

Full Heart Empty Womb

and having to be secretive about it. Any other medical condition you could be more open about going in for this test or treatment. Infertile people do not have that ability usually. It certainly adds to the stress level!

I had my ultrasound done by a substitute tech. Before then almost all of my ultrasounds had been done by the same tech, which was comforting. The new person had a very difficult time doing my ultrasound. Now, I will take part of the blame. I have been told that my uterus is tilted and is hard to read. Would you expect anything less from me? However, this ultrasound was downright painful. I was close to yelling, "It really will not go any further!! You are looking at my uterus not my lungs!"

I felt better though when I saw the results. My follicle appeared to have grown. This was a good sign. My hope was starting to grow again. Jordan told me she hated to have me come again but she felt like the next day may be the day that I was ready. She had also talked to Dr. Whitworth about using a drug called Neupogen® on me. Neupogen® is actually a drug that is used with cancer patients. It has been used in fertility treatments to help thicken a patient's endometrium.

I was on cloud nine when I walked out. My follicle was growing. The fluid was almost gone. I had ordered the Neupogen® that could help my lining thicken more. Everything was moving in the right direction. Maybe we wouldn't be cancelled after all! I figured out when the transfer would be so I could get child-care in place just in case. It was going to be the following Wednesday. There was a mother-son kickball tournament that day. I talked to my friend, Ginger, and she was ready to help out so that Ethan wouldn't be left out at all. Ella had a Daisy Scout meeting. I got my friend, Devon, to help with that. I talked to Windy about time I would need off work and she was supportive. I was so grateful that I had a few people with whom I could be open and from whom I could receive help!

Full Heart Empty Womb

On Wednesday I drove to NFC listening to praise music. I had tears of gratitude in my eyes. I felt like God was right there with me. I felt down to my bones that I was going to get pregnant. I just *knew* I would! I thanked Him for giving me the peace of mind. I didn't know if it was a defense mechanism to just get through another appointment or if it was truly God-given. Regardless, I was grateful to have peace in a very non-peaceful time.

Well, my appointment was horrible. When they measured my follicle, it appeared to have shrunk instead of grown. Since my ultrasound was so difficult the day before, I think that it was not measured correctly. The lining of my endometrium still wasn't good. It appeared that one of three things happened: 1. I had already ovulated = cancelled cycle because we missed the window despite our efforts. 2. I wasn't going to ovulate at all = cycle would be cancelled. This seemed to be the most likely, or 3. The small chance that I was ovulating late. They asked me to come back a fifth time on Thursday to see which of the three happened.

I sat in the little room struggling to hold back my tears. I hate to cry at all but I really hate to cry with people I don't know that well. I wished that I had asked Eric to come to the appointment with me! I could tell that Jordan's heart was breaking for me, too. She had a new nurse that was training with her. I can only imagine what that nurse's thoughts were.

I was devastated. My hopes had been so high just an hour before. I cried and cried the whole way to the kids' school to volunteer. I prayed and pulled myself together before I went in to their elementary school. I was sitting in the 1st grade hallway and inventorying Ethan's teacher's science kit and praying. I said, "Lord I understand that you have your own timeline. And I truly want your perfect will and plan for our life. I just don't understand. If I was going to be cancelled, then why wait until now? It could have been Friday, Monday, or Tuesday. But now? After I had my hopes up and I had made all these **plans**..." Immediately God said, "Jeremiah 29:11" in my head. It was the memory verse that I was helping the kids memorize that week. I

117

thought it was a good verse for new Christians to learn. And apparently me too! He said, "Stephanie, for **I** know the **plans** I have for you, **plans** to prosper you and <u>not harm you</u>, plans to give you hope and a future." Immediately I was at peace. I knew that God had us wrapped up in His arms and had the perfect plan for us. I just had to find peace in it and be patient.

Like it's my J-o-b

Cute sidebar story that will make sense in a few....

The Sunday before, the 1st graders were given Bibles at our church. Ethan and Ella were so excited to "read" through them on the way home. "Reading" to them was to flip through each of the books as quickly as they could. When Ethan got to the book of Job, he kept pronouncing it with a short o instead of a long o. We tried to explain to him that the book of the Bible was pronounced with a long o. He proceeded to mispronounce it repeatedly at least 20 times in 10 minutes. Eric and I gave up and just laughed. Later that day, I told him to get his reader to practice his reading. His book was about Ben the mailman. He read that Ben's job (**LONG O!!!**) was to deliver the mail! It was hysterical. So we'd had an ongoing joke about Job all week.

Now back to our regularly scheduled program…

Although I had a peace deep down, being human, I still found myself getting pulled back down with the "woe is me's" throughout Wednesday. What was tomorrow's ultrasound going to tell us? Fortunately, I had God's words to which I could cling. While I was making the kids dinner on Wednesday night I got pulled down again. I thought, "Lord why? Why have we had so many obstacles?? And not just little ones, but big painful ones! That surgery was horrible! Why? Why? Why?" Then again I heard Him say, "Stephanie. This is your JOB." Now I am in no way comparing my situation to Job. Job lost his whole family and everything he had. But this is Satan again trying to take away my joy that God gave to me. My peace that God gave to me. I just had to decide to not let Satan do that. Immediately it was lifted from me and I felt joy and hope again.

As I laid in bed Wednesday night, I praised God for the peace I had in His plan. I told him that I trusted in His perfect plan and will for our lives. But being me, I added, "But Lord if there is any way for a miracle, please let us have one. I am just so tired. Pastor Sam said Sunday to ask for miracles and I know you can do it *if it is in your plan.*" I slept for a few hours and woke up and prayed the same prayer for a couple more hours before my appointment.

As I drove to NFC for the fifth ultrasound in less than a week, I felt like I was trapped in the movie "Groundhog Day." This time I had Eric by my side though. How would this one unfold? I went in for my ultrasound at peace. Praying for my miracle but at peace that God had this time in complete control. Eric held my hand, and we were ready to face this together. As the ultrasound tech did my ultrasound, she was completely astounded. My follicle had grown to the perfect size (over 3 mm of growth) overnight. My lining, which was practically nonexistent before, was PERFECT. It was 8mm thick, had no fluid at all, and was perfectly even. No fertility drug could have created this transformation - let alone in less than 24 hours. And I was not taking anything. It was completely and totally God. The ultrasound tech gave her report to my doctor. Dr. Whitworth left the surgery center to perform another ultrasound on me herself because the transformation was so astounding. As she looked at it, she was completely amazed. Everything was perfect. When I got my blood work back, my estrogen level had tripled overnight. I went from completely broken to perfect overnight. She said, "It is like a completely different person. You are night and day from yesterday." I told her that was because I had been on my hands and knees praying night and day since yesterday. It was a complete miracle. I felt so incredibly blessed and humbled that God was right there with me through it all. I thought I was on cloud nine the other day. That didn't even compare to the joy I was feeling.

Full Heart Empty Womb

The FET was scheduled for the next Thursday. I would be able to play in the mother-son kickball game and I was grateful. It would also be two days before Matthew's birthday party and a week before Ethan and Ella's seventh birthday. I would have plenty of wonderful things to occupy my time and thoughts!

A couple of days before the transfer I was watching my kids in their gymnastics class. I got a text from my friend, Devon, who was in another part of the complex watching her daughters. She asked me to meet her so that she could pray with me before the transfer. Devon was one of the few people in my kids' "school world" that knew what was going on. She was a great support to me when I needed help with the kids. The thought that she wanted to sit and pray with me for the transfer was very moving to me. We sat on a little bridge between the two buildings and she prayed for Eric, our totsicles, and me. Afterwards she shared a verse with me. It was Ecclesiastes 11:5 (NIV). "As you do not know the path of the wind, or how the body is formed in a mother's womb, so you cannot understand the work of God, the maker of all things." I had never read this scripture before but I loved it. Of course I focused on the part about a body being formed in a mother's womb more than anything!

We went into the transfer the following Thursday feeling hopeful and completely at peace with the situation. The miraculous events leading up to the FET had given fuel to our hope. We were sure that we were going to get pregnant. I had written down Ecclesiastes 11:5 on a small slip of paper and held it close to my heart through the whole transfer.

The transfer was textbook, and I was home on bed rest before I knew it. Eric got me a yummy lunch that I ate quickly and laid back flat. My hands immediately went to my belly as I assured my babies that I would take good care of them if they stuck around. I drifted in and out of sleep all day as I rubbed my belly and whispered to my sweet totsicles. All the while I was still holding the scripture in my hand.

I took it easy the next day, too and had a cartoon marathon with Matthew while Ethan and Ella were at school. The following day was

Full Heart Empty Womb

Matthew's birthday party. I was so glad that we decided to have it at a local gym and not at our house. We pretty much just had to show up and watch the kids have a blast. I was surprised to realize at the end of the party that I had gone a couple of stretches without thinking about if I was pregnant or not. I made up for it that night! I wondered if I had overdone it at Matthew's party. Eric made sure I didn't lift a single thing. I sat as often as I could. I knew I didn't but that didn't stop the guilt. I had to keep reminding myself that fertile people don't have sex then not move a muscle for two weeks. It was just another way that I was trying to take control of the situation through my actions – or my inactions in this case. I repeatedly had to remind myself that it was in God's hands not mine.

The next week was a busy week for me at the preschool. Windy was so good to make sure that I never overexerted. My co-teacher, Kelly, wouldn't let me lift one more finger than necessary. I loved going to school. Even though I was surrounded by children, it was a good distraction from worrying about if I was pregnant or not. If one of the teachers wasn't making me laugh, then one of the kids would. It was a sweet, sweet distraction from the stress.

We celebrated Ethan and Ella's 7th birthday and all of the many blessings that we had. When Eric and I sat back and thought about where we were eight years before, it brought me to tears. Eight years before I had just had my first lap and we were getting ready to do our first IUI. Never in a million years did we think we would come so far in our journey to become parents. Parents of three children. Two via IVF. One a complete miracle straight from God. And now, possibly one or two more children? Amazing. Never in my life would I have orchestrated my family like this. More proof that God's plan is better than Stephanie's.

The weekend before my beta test we were busy going from birthday party to birthday party. We concluded the weekend with Ethan's birthday party. He had his party at a laser chase place. He was so excited about it. It was great to watch him and all of his friends race around the course. Ella, of course, was in the midst of it all, giggling and having a ball. Ella and the boys. The kids would gang up together and try to catch Eric. He took no prisoners though. I think he was living out his secret desire to be cop. He hid behind walls and jumped out at the boys. It was fantastic.

I floated around, watched, and tried to take pictures as the chaos ensued around me. I found Matthew looking sad in a corner. The poor little thing was weighed down by his oversized vest. He was crying because he was having a hard time playing. I debated for a minute and then chastised myself. My beta test was the next day. Seriously, I could carefully play one round of laser tag with a bunch of six and seven year olds and be ok. If the embryo(s) had implanted at all, then they had by this point. Again, fertile people don't sit around and do nothing! I gave myself a pep talk. "I am not being irresponsible. This is in God's hands not mine."

I wiped my baby's tears and put on his vest. Hand in hand we worked our way through the maze. He giggled with glee with each person he hit. I knew I made the right decision. Jordan had said some physical activity was ok. I didn't even break a sweat. It wasn't fair that I had to weed through so much guilt to get to it though.

That night I laid in bed with my hands on my belly singing and talking to my totsicles. I was so excited to have my beta the next day. I would not even let my mind drift to the possibility of my not being pregnant. I knew I was. I didn't have the first symptom, but I didn't let it get me down. Last time I had strong symptoms and I wasn't pregnant. It was just the side effects of the progesterone. This time I wasn't on progesterone, so I didn't feel anything. When I got pregnant with Ethan and Ella, I didn't feel much this early either. I fell asleep with happy tears going down my face onto my pillow with my hands laying on my belly.

The Last Beta

I made my last drive to NFC the next morning. I had my blood drawn just like I had countless times before. Matthew and I busied ourselves for the next few hours while we waited for Eric to come home. He was going to take a half day so that we could call and get the results together. I was so proud that I waited to call my voicemail until after lunch. What patience I had learned through all of this! The first time we called there wasn't a message. We decided to call every 15 minutes until we got a message. It was the longest afternoon of my life. I tried to carry on like normal with Matthew, but I had to run back to my room for privacy to make a call every time I turned around. I started to get nervous when it was almost time to pick up the big kids from school. By then it had been two and a half hours. Eric and I headed back to our room to make the call one last time before we went to pick them up.

"You have one new message," came over my speakerphone. We giggled and bounced up and down on the bed. This was it! Jordan's voice began, "Hi Stephanie, its Jordan. I am so sorry but I do not have good news for you today. The level came back negative. This is not what I was hoping for or expecting, and I know you must be devastated. I'm so sorry. Dr. Whitworth has not had a chance to review this, but when she does she will obviously be disappointed as well. When you are ready, I will arrange a time for you and Dr. Whitworth to talk about this so she can express condolences and discuss the cycle. If there is anything I can do for you please let me know."

If I had been standing, I would have fallen to my knees. The tears were immediate, falling fast down my cheeks. Eric was crying, too and he grabbed me and pulled me into a hard hug. The quiet tears turned to a gut-wrenching sob. "No. No. No!!! I just knew that I was pregnant." Eric wiped my tears and told me that he was just as sure that I was pregnant. We sat on our bed, crying and clinging to each other. I wished I could go back to an hour ago when I didn't know. When I had hope. When I thought our baby was in my belly.

Eric volunteered to go pick up the kids from school so that I could have some time to pull myself together. I was so grateful. I didn't feel like I could face anyone at that point. My phone continued to buzz as it had all day. Another text from a well-intentioned friend wanting to know if I heard anything or sending their support. I quickly sent a text and email to those that I had told. I turned off my phone and computer so I could escape the constant buzzing and dinging. I was grateful for all the support, but at that time I wished that no one else knew.

Eric got home with the kids and I hugged them fiercely. I blinked back the tears as I thought about their baby brother or sister that might have been. I went through the motions that night until bedtime. When it was time to say our prayers, I felt my heart ache. I gave the quickest, most generic prayer I could muster. It was hard for me. I wasn't exactly on speaking terms with God at that moment.

Once the kids were in bed, Eric told me to take a hot bath. I loved to take hot baths and was not able to do that after the embryo transfer. I filled the tub full of the hottest water I could stand and sank into my personal oasis. I closed my eyes and let the tears fall that I had bottled up for the last few hours. I put my hands on my empty womb and cried for the babies that I knew in my heart that I was going to have.

I cried for Amy Lynn. I cried for Noah. I cried for Charlotte and Nolan. Every one of them were real and my babies in my mind. I knew that I wouldn't get pregnant with all four, but I really thought I would get pregnant with at least one. After the dramatic and miraculous events with my lining prior to the transfer, I really thought that it was a sign that we would get pregnant.

I stayed in the bath until the water turned cold. I dried off, got dressed, and went to be with Eric. I curled on his lap and continued to cry. They were sad tears that were grieving the babies I would never know.

Then they turned to angry tears. I was mad at God. Why? We prayed about everything. Every decision that we made we prayed about first. He wanted us to pursue the FETs instead of embryo adoption. We were obedient even though it was very difficult for us. If I wasn't going to get pregnant, then why did it have to be so drawn out? Why couldn't it be as simple as we thought it would be – two back-to-back cycles? No. I had to be tortured and even have my fallopian tubes removed in the process.

The surgery just really made me mad to think about. It was a huge deal. I went through a tremendous amount of pain. And now without fallopian tubes it really was impossible for me to ever get pregnant naturally again. The door wasn't just closed. It was slammed in my face.

When I was exhausted from all the crying I finally fell asleep. I woke up the next morning with my eyes almost swollen shut. My hands were on my belly out of habit. I scolded myself for holding my empty womb out of nothing more than a habit now. It wasn't needed. There was no one there, and there never would be.

I slathered on the eye cream, got ready for work, and then worked on getting the kids ready for school. The whole drive to work I was giving myself a pep talk to make it through the day without tears. I opened the door to the preschool. It displayed a birth announcement of a baby brother that had been born recently. I saw Windy as I walked the hall to my classroom. She gave me a hard hug but didn't say anything. She knew I was trying to keep my emotions under control. Kelly was waiting for me in our classroom. I had texted her the night before and told her not to hug me because I would lose it. But I decided I needed it. I dropped my bag and went straight to her for a warm hug.

It was a long day. The kids made me laugh and forget my sadness for a while. Then I would see a mom that was expecting. Or one of the teachers would start talking about something to do with her babies. Being in a preschool was like being in a torture chamber. I was grateful for the few there that did know so that I could get support from them when I needed it.

When we got all our babies down for a nap, I went to Windy's office. I knew Windy would be a good person to talk to about things. She understood infertility intimately. She had prayed me through the last couple of years. We sat in her office, and she let me unload, and she cried with me. It was just what I needed. I didn't need anyone to rationalize my situation. I just needed someone to listen to me and agree that it wasn't fair.

The next day I was cleaning the playroom when I heard my phone ring. My heart skipped a beat when I saw "NFC" on my caller ID. I answered the phone tentatively and heard Dr. Whitworth on the other end of the line. She told me how very sorry she was that it didn't work. She told me that she was very hopeful for Eric and me. I gave her one of my several canned answers I had ready to go, assuring her I was ok. She asked if we were interested in pursuing another IVF. I tried to explain where my head was. "We decided to do the FET because we wanted *those* embryos. *Those* babies that we helped create seven years ago. We wanted *those* babies. We loved *those* babies. We had a responsibility to *those* babies. We didn't want just any baby. We wanted *those* babies. I cannot even imagine going through the pain of IVF again." She said she completely understood and wished me the best of luck.

Chapter Seven – My Unique Grief

I didn't realize it at the time but I went through the whole grieving process for my babies. The first stage is denial. I did not deny that I was not pregnant. I was painfully aware that I was not then, nor would I ever be, pregnant again. After I had a couple of good days of crying, I was in denial that I was upset. "I can't be upset. How can I be sad? I have three beautiful children. I have no right to be sad", I thought. Ethan, Ella, and Matthew were a wonderful reminder to me of all the blessings that I have been given. I was enormously grateful for the children I had. When I was sad I could always wrap one of them up in a big hug and snuggle them until the threat of tears passed. Then I immediately felt shame for the sadness. The pain, the loss that I felt was real, but I felt like I was not allowed to feel it.

When people asked how I was doing, I had several responses ready to go. "Of course we are sad, but we are so grateful for the many blessings that God has given us." Or, "It was a hard year, but we are grateful for how much closer it has made us." Or, "Really! I am fine! I am sure why we went through all this will make sense to me someday!"

One day I went up into our attic to get some longer pants out for our kids. We had a good cold snap and all the kids were wearing high-water pants to school! I was fortunate to have lots of hand-me-down clothes from my sister and sister-in-law. When I got up to the top, I was assaulted by the bins and bins of baby clothes that I had saved for our babies. I had at least 12 bins full of clothes. I also had baby toys and other things that I knew we would use again. I teared up a bit as I questioned how we would have a baby to use any of it.

When I got down from the attic I picked up the phone and called my sister-in-law, Amy, and told her about my grand plan. We were going to have one stinking big garage sale. I was going to sell it all, get it out of my house, and use the proceeds to buy my babies a new swing set. They had outgrown the one we had now and we were just holding on to it for the baby. Well, that wasn't needed now. Amy was excited to hop on board with me. We made plans to have it the following Saturday. We were even going to get the kids to sell hot chocolate. Who can resist cute kids selling hot chocolate on a cold day?

Eric went out of town that week for work. After I put the kids to bed, I spent every night tagging clothes and toys. I would reminisce a little bit as I picked up some of my favorite outfits. So many good memories. I had so much for which to be grateful. I was actually excited as I got things together for the garage sale. We had so much stuff that we actually could make enough to get the kids a new swing set! Denial. It wasn't until I got to the box of newborn clothes that it hit me. I pulled out tiny sleepers, gowns, little hats and bibs and the tears came hard and fast again. No baby. You saved all of this for nothing.

The garage sale was a success. We sold most everything and loaded the rest up to be donated. None of it was coming back into my house. The kids sold their hot chocolate and felt accomplished as they counted out the dollars they earned.

Eric's surgery was quickly approaching. We made arrangements yet again for the kids. They would alternate between my parents and Eric's so that I could stay in the hospital with him. I literally typed out a four page Word document with all the details about the kids' schedule, school, and anything else I could think of for our parents while I was gone. I didn't have time to sit around and mope. I still cried some at night when I let my thoughts wander.

Eric had a foot of his colon removed in mid-November. Everything went exactly as expected and we were grateful for a smooth surgery. My dad came in to his room and made a joke asking Eric if he now had a semicolon. Eric gave a laugh then winced because it hurt too much to laugh. It was a long, hard five days in the hospital for Eric. He got up, and we walked the halls as often as he was able.

As much as I hated the circumstances, I was grateful to repay Eric in a small way for him taking care of me so much. I laid each night on the very uncomfortable recliner chair. I wondered how in the world Eric did it for me for so long. 77 nights he slept like this by my side. He never complained once.

He slept a lot because of his pain meds, so I was left with my own thoughts a lot. I remembered that when we had thought about managing his hospital stay, we thought that I would be pregnant. I had wondered if I would have morning sickness. I thought I would have to pack plenty of lemon drops to help soothe my tummy! At least now I could give 100% of myself to help him recuperate. That was true, of course, but I was in denial. I would have loved nothing more than to be sick as a dog in the hospital bathroom.

Occasionally Eric and I talked about things. I tried not to talk about it too much because I didn't want to put any more stress on him. Usually it was about some of the stress that was not in our life because I wasn't pregnant. Like, "Well at least we don't have to worry about moving to a different house!" or "Hey, we may just be able to afford to go to Disney World again now!" or "Wow, I will have some free time when Matthew starts Kindergarten." Denial. I would have gladly moved if it meant we had another child to make room for. Disney World? Who needs Disney World if we have another baby? We can have fun in our backyard! Free time? I haven't had free time in seven years. What would I like to do most in my free time? Love on a baby. It didn't matter how much "easier" things were for us. I would have rather things be more chaotic and had my baby to love and hold.

Full Blown ANGER

By the time Eric went to his two week post op appointment with his surgeon, he was doing great. His age and good health had really helped him heal quite well. He had been to see the same surgeon a couple of years before for a hernia that he was supposed to get repaired. He never did because it didn't bother him enough to deal with it. At his follow up appointment, he joked that after all our medical bills this year he would really like to squeeze in his hernia surgery before the end of the year. Between his knee surgery, our FETs, my surgery, and now his colon surgery, we had sailed past our deductible.

I was surprised when he let us schedule his surgery. It was set for a week before Christmas. It was "just a lap surgery" so we expected a long weekend kind of recovery. You would think after my last lap surgery that we would have learned our lesson! He had the surgery and it went well. The recovery, however, was horrible. I think it was because he was still getting over his first surgery. If he had been 100% before the surgery, then his recovery would have been smoother.

Eric felt horrible. Christmas is his favorite time of year. He loves everything about it. Shopping for the kids' Christmas presents is something he enjoys more than anything. Instead he was stuck in his recliner alternating between heat and ice.

Between taking care of Eric and getting ready for Christmas, I was running full speed from sun up to sun down and beyond. All the while I was stuffing my emotions, my grief, and my pain deep down. I didn't have time to deal with it. I had to take care of Eric. I had to take care of the kids. We were going out of town for a week so I had to get us all packed. I had to get ready for Christmas for the whole family all by myself.

One night when I was working on sending out our Christmas cards and was beyond exhausted, the dam broke. When I thought I was going to be pregnant, I had a cute Christmas card all planned out that would announce my pregnancy. I cried. I yelled. I believe I may have even stomped my feet. All the while Eric looked on in fear from his recliner thinking my head may actually start to spin. I was ANGRY. I wanted my baby! I had four embryos. Why couldn't I have one of them? Why did the road have to be so hard and so painful? If God knew we weren't going to get pregnant then why drag it out? We could have done the two FETs back to back like we had planned. Every day that passed I fell more and more in love with the baby that I *knew* waited for me at the end of the journey. A baby that I would never know.

Bargaining

It is hard not to second guess the decisions that you make. When you are going through fertility treatments, you make tons of decisions at every turn. Eric and I took every decision we had to make and prayed over them until we felt God's direction for us. This prayer helped me a lot through the "bargaining" stage of grief. I would certainly think from time to time, "What if I took all the drugs the last time?" or "Maybe we should have waited." Then I would always remember that we prayed about it and did what God wanted us to do. That is a peace that you can only get from God.

Depression

During Christmas I went from angry to just depressed. I kept thinking about how excited we were the year before. We just knew that we were going to have a baby (or two!) by this time. I remember we stayed up late watching cheesy Lifetime Christmas movies because "we wouldn't be able to do that next year with a newborn!"

I worked very hard to keep up my façade during the day with the kids and the rest of my family. At night I would cry myself to sleep. I felt so alone in my grief. What happened a couple of months ago with our failed FET wasn't even on anyone's radar screen but mine. Eric was sad but he had come to accept it. And my family just didn't understand. Mostly that was my fault because I never talked about it. I didn't want to bring everyone down. So I smiled and acted like everything was fine when I was crumbling inside.

Full Heart Empty Womb

I remember one day crying to the point that I could hardly catch my breath. I called my mom when I calmed down a bit. I asked her to pray for me and she asked, "Why? What is wrong?" She had no idea that I was still struggling with my grief so much. I felt so alone, but I didn't have to be. I had to reach out and let some people know I needed help.

That is where this is tricky. When you are grieving a person, everyone knows. There is a funeral for you to say a symbolic goodbye. You have a visitation where friends and family can offer their condolences and support. They may even bring you a casserole for those days when you don't even think you can get out of bed. I was going through the entire grieving process almost completely in a vacuum. On the outside I was still the smiling preschool teacher and happy mama. Few people even knew what happened. And no one understood the pain that I went through that continued to linger in my life.

One Sunday morning after I had a particularly bad night, I told Eric to just take the kids to church without me. I couldn't put on the mask that morning. I didn't have the energy to pretend. With sad eyes, he agreed to take them without me. I got dressed and worked out. Then I took my time taking a shower and making out my grocery list. It was a leisurely morning and I loved it. As I was walking down the empty aisle of the grocery store I thought, "This is nice! I should spend every Sunday morning like this." Instantly I felt shame. No. This is not who I wanted to be. I was hurt, angry, and sad but I had to find a way to get past it. I could not turn my back on God.

That was a real turning point for me. I got an appointment with a counselor at the church to help me talk through some things. He affirmed that I was going through the grieving process. He really validated it for me, too. I desperately needed that. I needed to hear from someone that it was ok that I was grieving. This grief was a completely unconventional situation, but I was going through real emotions and pain.

I wish that I could say that at that turning point things instantly turned around for me, but it took effort. I made myself start praying more. After I had my negative pregnancy test, my time in prayer dropped dramatically. For the most part the only time I prayed was with the kids before bed, and it was halfhearted to say the least.

I started having some quiet time in the morning. I usually did it in the shower so that the water and tears would mix down my face. I got very raw and real with God. I talked about my pain and my anger. It didn't go away, but it lessened a little each day.

Acceptance

In many ways, going through the grieving process in my vacuum is what gave me the motivation to write this book. I have never felt as alone in my whole life as I did that year. I was surrounded by people who loved me but they just didn't understand what I was going through. I don't think you can understand unless you go through it yourself.

I honestly did not really get to the point of acceptance until a year passed. It took me a while to get through all the emotions and be able to think things through a little more rationally. The next chapter digs a little deeper into what I learned through my acceptance.

Chapter Eight – A Little Monday Quarterbacking

If you can't already tell, I will let you in on a secret. I am not a writer. However, all my life I have sort of narrated in my head. Eric would say that proves my craziness. I would say that I like to tell a good story. I am not sure if "good" is the right adjective for my story, but I think it is a story worth telling.

I started blogging a bit after I had Ethan and Ella. It was a good way to update the family about how they were doing. I also loved to share all the funny, cute stories they gave me. Many days I felt like I lived in a sitcom. If I could bring a smile to someone's face with something I said, it made my day. Around the time I had Matthew, I was introduced to this new (at least to me) phenomenon called Facebook. I loved it! I could post pictures without stressing about spacing and layout. And there was no pressure to write a long essay. Hooray!!! So long! Away went my blog into a cyber-cemetery.

All along my journey through infertility, I felt a little nudge from God to tell my story. Even in the high drama of my high-risk pregnancy with Ethan and Ella, I was skeptical. What was so different and special about my story? I remember having a stronger nudge when I was going through the fertility treatments in 2013. I would think, "If I get pregnant, then that would make a good story and I will write it." Or, "If I get pregnant with twins again, then that would make for a *really good* story and I will tell it." I had all these ideas of what needed to happen for my story to be worth telling. I struggled for a while over whether I should write my story and wondered if I really had anything worth telling.

In the midst of my struggle, I had a good friend that suffered a great tragedy with one of her children. When I heard, I was just devastated for her. I thought, "How in the hell can I complain about anything that I have suffered in comparison to her pain?" I swear to you I heard

God say to me, "Stephanie. Just because her pain may be different and even greater, that does not make your pain any less ***valid and real***." That solidified my resolve once and for all that my story, our stories, of infertility deserve to be told. We deserve to be understood. You need to know that YOU ARE NOT ALONE.

I feel as though I need to state before I dive into it that this narrative is written with infertility firmly in my rearview mirror. I certainly didn't have this clarity in the midst of it. Some of it is much easier said than done. However, all are things that I wish someone had talked to me about. I may have shook my head and said, "Yeah, right. Easier said than done." But a seed would have been planted and I would have at least seen things from a different perspective. I had books and doctors that told me what I needed to do to try to get pregnant. I had nothing that told me how to take care of my heart and mental stability in the process.

Why Me??

A question that continually went through my mind during my infertility journey was, "Why me?" It seemed like everyone around me was getting pregnant just by thinking about it. Why did I have to be different? What in the world was wrong with me? Why did God put this burning desire in my heart to be a mother, but make it impossible for me to get pregnant? It seemed so cruel.

I struggled with all those questions daily. After I did my last FET and the door was shut so firmly in my face, I grew very, very bitter. Not only did I not get pregnant with any of my sweet totsicles, but I lost my fallopian tubes. They're kind of necessary if those eggs had a prayer of getting to the sperm. And we know my eggs have to do all the work because Eric's sperm don't know where the hell to go! Why did God lead me down that road for just heartache? It took time and prayer for me to get to healing and a place of understanding.

Full Heart Empty Womb

Ladies, we all have rotten *stuff* that happens in our lives. Some lose a parent at a young age. Some suffer abuse. Some are afflicted with a disease or have a loved one that is. Some spend years of their life trying to become a mommy. No matter who you are, *stuff* happens. We are imperfect people living in an imperfect world.

I often wondered why God didn't just make it all go away and make me pregnant. I mean He is God, isn't He? Haven't I done everything right? I have been positive, upbeat, prayed daily. Hadn't I done what He wanted me to do? What was the magic formula or magic prayer that I had to say to make Him answer the prayer *the way I wanted Him to?*

Being a mother has given me a little bit of insight to help me understand why. As a mom, nothing makes me happier than when my children are happy. And nothing will make me sadder than to see my babies' tears.

Fortunately, we haven't had any big drama in our children's lives yet that we have had to endure. I can think back to my childhood and recall very distinctly a time when my parents had to watch me go through a tough time and allow me to learn and grow from it. When I was in high school I was a very shy girl. We had moved to Kentucky from Texas. It was a tough transition for me. Everyone at my new school had already formed their cliques. No one was really interested in letting the new girl in. I met a guy at church that showed interest in me. I mistook attention for love. We started dating and I spent every second I could with him. He was kind of arrogant and kind of a jerk, but I was blinded by my teenage love.

I learned my lesson, but unfortunately it came with a great deal of pain. When we went away to college, he turned emotionally abusive and violated my trust in the worst kind of way. I finally found my strength and broke up with him. When I did my parents were there for me with open arms.

It was an extremely tough time in my life. Through it I learned a lot of important lifelong lessons. I learned the value of self-respect. I learned that there should be mutual respect in a relationship. I learned that God never runs out of forgiveness for us. I also learned that although there is forgiveness, sometimes there are also still consequences for our mistakes. I learned the importance of finding the man that God had out there for me. I learned to cherish that man with every fiber of my being when I finally found him. All of these things were difficult to learn, but they are the bedrock of my strong marriage today - a marriage that not only survived infertility but *thrived* through infertility *twice*.

I believe that is what God experiences with us. All of this rotten stuff is an opportunity to learn and come out on the other side of it better and stronger. Through the tough times we can develop character. I know without a doubt that I would not be as good of a wife to Eric, mother to my children, and daughter to Christ had I not been through infertility.

Ladies, you have two choices: you can choose to be bitter, angry, and sad about your situation. And there certainly is a time and place for that! We are human. And honestly, being infertile is unfair! I have written pages upon pages about the pain that it took for us to get pregnant. For the vast majority of the world, it just takes a romantic evening! But hopefully you can make a decision to move to the second choice; you can choose to learn and grow from the situation and come out on the other side a better person. If you make a conscious effort, I am sure you will see that there is a lot in your life for which to be grateful. Try not to lose focus on those things with which you are blessed. You may not even be able to get to the second choice for a long time. Praying about it can help you get there. You may even bounce between the two. Just don't let yourself camp out on being bitter and angry forever.

Because there are also two absolutes. You may feel the after effects for a while, but the painful road of infertility will come to an END. The choice you make may or may not affect whether you have a baby or not but it will affect YOU. Don't let infertility take anything else from you! It may have taken away your ability to get pregnant, but don't let it take away YOU.

You have already survived more than you ever thought you would on this road. You are strong. Continue to pray for strength and guidance with the many decisions you are faced with every single day. You can come through infertility stronger than you ever dreamed you would be.

Lean on Him

"All that is fine and good," I am sure you think. But how in the world do you do it?? Whether you have grown up going to church or have never stepped foot in a church, there is one thing I can say with complete certainty. God is there for you, and He wants you to lean on Him. Lean on Him? That is a phrase that we throw around in church a lot. We sing about it, we preach about it, we hug each other and tell you to lean on God. What does that even mean? Personally I love the mental picture that the phrase brings to mind. I see God in the typical illustrations in children's Bibles. Long flowing white robe, long brown hair, brown beard. A face with a kind smile and caring eyes. Ladies, He is always there right beside us. We just have to lean on Him to feel and see Him for the Rock that He is.

It brings to mind a time when Eric and I were in a fight. We had said our apologies, but I was still just sitting next to him on the couch pouting and being stubborn. He sat next to me and put his arm around me. I continued to sit still and stare at the TV and didn't acknowledge him. I still had some mad I needed to work out. Finally, I got over it and relaxed. I leaned into him. He tightened his arm around me and kissed me on top of the head. Then my floodgates opened. I started to cry and hugged him back. He picked me up, put me on his lap, and held me in a strong embrace. He smoothed my hair and told me repeatedly that he loved me.

Ladies, that is exactly what God will do for you. It is what He is sitting right next to you begging you to do. "Lean on me, child. Please. I am ready to pick you up, place you on my lap, and comfort you." When we let our floodgates open with God and lean on Him, we will feel His embrace, His presence with us. As I have said repeatedly in this book, you are not alone. God is right there beside you. All you have to do is just *lean*.

Power of Prayer

Aside from the obvious blessing of my children, my closer relationship with God has been the best blessing of infertility. In any healthy relationship you have to communicate. With God, one way is through prayer. As you can probably tell, I am a huge believer in the power of prayer. Sometimes that prayer is a long, drawn out, tear-filled plea. Sometimes it is a quick sentence to help dry your tears so you can just get out of your car. There are many times when I was talking to God that all I could get out was, "Please, Please, Please" as I rubbed my belly. He heard all those prayers.

My first trip through infertility, I will admit that probably 95% of my prayers revolved around just getting me pregnant. The second time around I certainly prayed about that a lot, too.

This summer my oldest son, Ethan, was determined to pass his swim test at the YMCA. Eric and I had spent a small fortune putting all the kids through swim lessons, so *we* were also determined for him to pass his swim test! Every time we went swimming, he would practice and practice. He took the test 4 times before he finally passed in the last few weeks of summer. He told me afterwards that he had been praying all summer about it. He said, "At first I prayed that God would go back in time and make me pass the test." Then he chuckled and said, "That didn't work out so well, so I changed what I was praying. I started to pray for confidence." Ethan learned a lot during those frustrating months of trying and failing. He learned to persevere. He learned to not give up. He learned that he had to work hard to get that reward.

I am not at all saying that you shouldn't pray to get pregnant. I am saying that there are a lot of things you can pray about that can help you on your journey. Here are some examples of additional things you can pray about to help you through your journey:

- God use infertility to bring my husband and me closer together.
- God please give me the strength I need to make it through this day.
- God please help me use this pain to help someone else. There are other infertile women that only you can help!
- God help me be patient.
- God please help us make the right decision.
- God please give me the peace about this situation.
- God please be with my family members and friends and help them be sensitive to my situation.
- God help me focus on the blessings in my life.

It is 100% completely natural to be angry and resentful about your infertility. You may find that it is just downright hard to pray because you are angry. After my failed FETs in 2013, I was very much just going through the motions in my prayer life. Pretty much the only time I prayed was either for Eric's comfort and healing or the nightly prayers with the kids. It wasn't until I had some time to heal and I realized I was on a path heading away from God that I made a change. God has big shoulders. He is omniscient and knows everything you are thinking and feeling whether you want to say it or not. Why not just lay it all out? Then ask Him to help change your heart. That is what I did. I told him that I was angry and felt betrayed, but I didn't want to be. I wanted to really be the way I was pretending to be. Over time He healed my broken heart.

I also think the amount of time that Eric and I spent in prayer helped us tremendously with all the decisions we had to make. When you are dealing with infertility, you have HUGE decisions facing you left and right. How do you make the right ones? And if things don't go your way, how do you deal with that? Because we prayed so much about each decision we made, God gave us a deep peace about the direction we went. After the heartache of last year, having the confidence that we definitely made the right decisions was priceless. There are no "what ifs" or "maybe we should haves." We know without a shadow of a doubt that we made the right decisions.

Hearing Him

A couple of times I was blessed to actually hear God talk right to me. No, there wasn't a burning bush or a thundering voice coming down from the Heavens. There were thoughts that were planted in my mind directly from God, which brought me comfort or understanding. My little mind did not have that depth of understanding on its own. The thoughts were divine. There were other ways in which God spoke to me throughout my journey. One day maybe it was a scripture that I came across. Another day maybe it was part of a sermon that seemed like it was directed straight at me. Maybe it was a song on the radio that gave me the encouragement I needed that day. Sometimes it was praise music but sometimes it was the Foo Fighters or Bon Jovi. I get daily devotionals sent to me. It is amazing how many times the subject line of the emails grabs me because it is exactly what I need to hear at that particular moment.

I highly recommend having a quiet time each morning. It doesn't have to be long. Just 20 minutes when you read a little devotional and spend some time in prayer with God asking for the strength to get through the day or to help you with the decisions you have to make. I think doing it in the morning is the best because it starts your day off on the right track. I think it also opens up your heart and mind to hear God speak to you throughout the day. Think of it as putting up your "antenna" for the day!

Along those same lines, in the morning at our house I have a rule. Only positive, uplifting music. I love music. I think the right music can lift your mood instantly. Sometimes it is contemporary Christian. Sometimes it is secular. It always is upbeat so that we can start our days off right. I cannot tell you how many times a song has come on the radio, and I felt like God had a message in it that He wanted me to hear. God wants to talk to you. You just have to be open to hear Him.

Take Care of YOU

Infertility is exhausting mentally and physically. It can seriously take its toll on your body. The hormones can cause you to gain weight. You go on and off of exercise and lifting restrictions depending on your treatment. It makes it very difficult to stay motivated with your fitness. I encourage you to find some way to stay active. Being active just makes you feel better. You don't have to do an hour-long kickboxing class to be active. You can go for a leisurely walk around the block. Take a yoga class. You can even just do some light stretching while you watch TV at night. All of these things will make you feel better physically and emotionally. Being active can help your stress level tremendously. Talk to you doctor. I am sure there is something that you can agree on that maintains the restrictions but also gives you the needed physical activity. I was pleasantly surprised at how much the restrictions had lessened between my first round of fertility treatments and the second.

Don't lose sight of your hobbies. Taking the time to enjoy your hobbies can be a much needed distraction. They can also be quite gratifying. Hobbies can remind you that there is more to your life than your journey to becoming a mother. I love to read. I could spend hours in an imaginary world and escape from my worries for at least a little while. Of course I had to be careful about my book selection! And on the flip side, writing in a journal about your journey may be a great deal of help for you, too. Sometimes writing things down helps you work through your feelings.

If you don't have a hobby, this is a great time to try to find one. It is an opportunity to have another positive goal in your life. You could also look for volunteer opportunities. Volunteering can be a wonderful way to relieve stress. You can help others, and I promise you will be blessed in the process, too. It can redirect your thoughts if only for the time you are there. You will probably find that there are a lot of areas in your life that you are very grateful for that have been covered by the infertility haze.

If you have children and are dealing with Secondary Infertility, you have some unique challenges. Let people help you with your children. If someone is gracious enough to offer to help watch them, then take them up on it! Whether it is for a doctor's appointment or just so you can take a moment to catch your breath.

Don't get pulled into the trap of feeling like you have to have play dates, be on every ball team, and help out at the school all the time. Our kids are overbooked today. That adds a tremendous amount of stress on you. I had all three of my kids playing on three different ball teams during my first FET. That was six games and practices each week. Only one of them really even wanted to play. This horrible "Mommy Guilt" makes you feel like you have to do everything and you don't. Think back to when you were little. We didn't require a fraction of what kids today do. Give yourself and your kids permission to take it easy.

My last bit of advice may sound a little silly but I swear to you it helps. When you go through infertility treatments the hormones, lack of physical activity, and stress can be hell on your body. If you aren't at least a little bloated, then you are really lucky. In between my last surgery and my last FET, I just went and bought a couple of pairs of pants a size up. The way I saw it either I would be pregnant and need them larger or I would just be more comfortable where I was. If I wore clothes that felt comfortable then I just felt better.

Protect your Marriage

It is so easy to put your life on hold when you are dealing with infertility. Eric and I did that a lot. It is one thing I would really change if I could go back. Not because I wish we had gone to this exotic place or that. I wish we had taken the time to focus just on us. You don't have to get on a plane. Stay in the Holiday Inn on the other side of town. The whole point is that you get out of your regular environment and focus on your marriage. It is so important that you protect your marriage when going through infertility. You don't know if you are going to be on this road for a year or five years. It can tear your marriage apart if you give it even a foothold. Take a weekend and just focus on each other and why you love each other so much. Even if it is just going out to dinner and making it a "No Infertility Discussion Allowed!!" time. If you don't have a strong marriage, then you can't be strong parents for sure!

Eric and I also went to couples fertility counseling. The decision was one of the best we ever made. It is also where I met my lovely editor, Rachael, and her husband, Jason. I learned a lot through that counseling. One of the things I learned about was the difference in how men's minds work. They are much better at compartmentalizing things in their mind. For us, that meant that it was easier for Eric to be able to lock away the "infertility" subject than it was for me. For me, it was always on my mind. There was no locking it away by any means! I could talk about what we were going through from the moment he got home from work to the moment our heads hit the pillow. Our counselor, Sheryl, suggested that we allot a certain amount of time to talk about our infertility and when that time was done, we were done talking about it. I know it sounds crazy. It was written in my Franklin Planner, "7:00 pm – Infertility discussion with Eric." It was good for both of us though. It gave Eric a breather from my incessant ramblings and tears. For me, it gave me a dedicated time that he *had* to talk to me about it. It also forced me to let it go and not focus on it all the time. Time's up! Now we need to do something to get my mind off infertility.

Allow your husband to be a part of your treatments as much as possible. If he can come to the appointments, then ask him to. You will never regret having his support there. If he can help you with your injections, then allow him to do them. Looking back I wish I had gotten Eric to do them our second round. I wasn't trying to keep him from it. I was just being practical. I could do the injections real quick before everyone got up, and we could be on with our day. I never asked him to come to doctor appointments because there were too many and he needed to be at work. I think if I had let him do the shots or asked him to come to a few appointments, he would have felt more a part of the process. I certainly wouldn't have felt so alone if I had allowed him to be more active in our journey.

Surround Yourself with Good Friends

A common mistake that a lot of infertile woman make is to hang their head in shame and not tell anyone. I am not saying that you need to make it your status update on Facebook. But you need someone to talk to about what you are going through or it will eat you alive. It is a balancing act for sure. You also need to keep in mind that every person you tell will also be someone that will want an update from you. Sending that mass email after my last failed FET was painful.

When I first found out I was infertile, I was in my late twenties. My friends were just starting to get pregnant, and I was the only one having problems. That made it very difficult to talk to my friends about it. I literally was the only one so none of them really knew much about it. They just knew that I made them uncomfortable. They didn't know what to say and what *not* to say. I was extremely fortunate to have my best friend, Jodi. I know it was tough on her because she was pregnant with her first child, Bryce, and had no experience with infertility. She never knew what to say but she never gave up trying. When in doubt she would just let me cry and say, "That sucks." And that was usually what I needed to hear. There was no rationalizing it away.

I found that I needed people who knew what I was going through to talk to though. I found a group of seven ladies on an internet support group that quickly became my lifeline. We were all so different. Different religions (from Baptist, to Mormon, to Wiccan, to Atheist) from all over the US (from Boston to California) and all different infertility issues (male factor, PCOS, unexplained). But we were drawn together because we all longed to be a mother. We were all at various stages of fertility treatments. We checked in with each other constantly. We cheered for each other. Prayed for each other. Cried for each other because we all knew exactly what the others were going through. Unless you have been through infertility, you really do not understand it. It is so important to find someone to talk to that understands what you are going through and can support you.

When I went through my second round of fertility treatments, my life was different. I had drifted away from that online infertility group for a few reasons. I was friends with all of my close friends from there on Facebook so I could keep up with them there. I was incredibly busy so going to one place to catch up with my various circles of friends was awesome. Also, I just wanted to leave the world of infertility behind. I didn't want a constant reminder of the pain I went through. I was ready to move on. Little did I know that I couldn't move on for a while.

Very few people knew that we were going through fertility treatments in 2013. I was very fortunate to have a solid group of girl friends that I could talk to. Unfortunately, as we got older more and more of my friends were faced with fertility issues. Those same girls that were with me the night I met Eric in 1998? They helped pray me through 2013.

Full Heart Empty Womb

I also had a good group of ladies from my Sunday school class that came to a book club at my house every couple of weeks. My friend, Amanda, and I started the book club when we were stressed about our oldest babies starting Kindergarten. Looking back it is amazing to see how God knit our group together. Over the last couple of years, every one of us has dealt with infertility or loss at one time or another. He knew that we could be there for each other like no other could be.

It helped that I had a person or two that knew what was going on in the various environments in which I spent most of my time. My director of the preschool, Windy, was and is my biggest champion. She was incredibly understanding about the time off that I had to take. My co-teacher, Kelly, gave me a hug when I needed it and made me laugh when I wanted to forget about it for at least a little while. At the kids' elementary school, I had a handful of friends that helped me in a lot of ways. My co-room mom, Melissa, was completely understanding and helped pick up my slack when I had conflicting appointments. Ginger was ready to jump in and be Ethan's mom, too at the mother-son kickball tournament if I missed. Devon was ready to take my kids home if I had a late appointment. All of these things helped me as I was working through the chaos of juggling kids, teaching, and infertility treatments. But the most important thing they did for me was pray for me. They were there to give me an encouraging hug or smile when I felt beat down. You don't have to go through this alone!

If you don't have a friend in your life that you are comfortable talking to about it, then do not despair! Look into infertility counseling. Go find an online support group. www.resolve.org is the website for the National Infertility Association. It is a wealth of information and support for infertile people. Finally, pray that God sends that special someone to help support you. He hears your prayers!

Permission to Protect

Research has shown that the level of stress that an infertile person goes through during fertility treatments is comparable to the stress of a person suffering from a serious illness. That is staggering to me. After living through it, I can say with 100% confidence that it is true. You also have the added burden that you are suffering in silence. There are no meals being brought to your family to help out when you are suffering. There are no cards or flowers that are sent for you to "Get pregnant soon!" You do not get the support that others who are going through this amount of stress are given.

That being said, if there is anything that you can do to limit or eliminate a source of stress, then you must do it. Baby showers? You have a free pass to miss every one. Catch a cold. Have other plans. Whatever. Do not put yourself through that torture. Eric and I went to a couples baby shower of some dear friends of ours shortly after I got pregnant with Ethan and Ella. I overheard Eric talking to one of his friends that also had problems with infertility. They were talking about how hard baby showers were for their wives. Eric adamantly said that if I were not pregnant then we would have had to miss the shower. It warmed my heart so much that he understood. I also realized that it would have been just as hard for him, but the men in our lives are forced to deal with it as often. Protect your heart.

If there are certain friends or acquaintances that are insensitive to your infertility, then limit your time with them if you even have to see them at all. Family members are a bit trickier. I think you need to be open with your immediate family about your struggles and your feelings. If you have a hard time expressing it yourself, then maybe share with them some excerpts from this book. I think even people who aren't infertile can read about my journey and hopefully get a more sympathetic view of infertility. You don't need any more stress in your life. You need to surround yourself with encouraging people that can help you cope through this difficult time.

If you have some flexibility at work, try not to take on any big projects when you know that you are going to be cycling. I know I terribly overcommitted myself at the kids' school in 2013. That was stress that I put on myself! I didn't have to do any of what I signed up to do. I should have given myself a free pass until I was done with the fertility treatments. It wasn't like I was the only mom in the school and things wouldn't get done if Stephanie Greer didn't sign up!

The Forks on Infertility Road

In the aftermath of the failed fertility treatments in 2013, I went through an angry, bitter phase. I asked God why it had to be so hard. Why did it have to be so painful? Why couldn't I have just done the two cycles quickly like I planned? Why did the pain have to be drawn out over a year and end with me not even getting pregnant? I felt like God had turned His back on me. I had been obedient. I had been faithful. Why was I in so much pain?

It honestly has taken me to this very day to start to understand. Literally this morning it dawned on me. The pain that I went through in 2013 was not only because I am infertile but because of the choice that we made when we faced that fork on the Infertility Road.

Bear with me here as I explain. In 2005 when we were in the midst of our infertility struggle, we prayed and prayed about what steps to take. We decided to pursue fertility treatments. We felt completely at peace with that decision. That was the fork on the road that God led us to take. He blessed us on that path through my pregnancy with Ethan and Ella. I will ***never*** regret that decision.

There are other forks on the Infertility Road that you can take. Each fork has its own unique challenges, pain and heartache. I never thought I would be strong enough to handle all of the possible heartaches that could come with the adoption process. If God had wanted us to adopt then I firmly believe He would have changed my heart. He would have given me the confidence I needed to tackle the overwhelming process. If we had taken the fork on the road where we chose to accept that we couldn't be parents, we would have had heartache, too. Lifelong heartache as we watched our friends' children grow, knowing we would never have the same. Unfortunately sometimes you don't get to pick the fork on the road, it is chosen for you after you get a detour from another.

However, when you decide to go down the path of fertility treatments, it is important to understand the hard road that you are going to take. Yes, you will have a chance to get pregnant when you may not have the chance on your own. I thank God for blessing us with the medical advances that allow infertile people the opportunity to become pregnant, too.

You also open yourself up to experience more pain and stress than cycling on your own. When you are going through infertility treatments you have so much more information about what is going on in that very complicated body of yours. Often times that is a wonderful thing that allows the doctors to put you on the right drug protocol that improves your chances to get pregnant. Other times it tells you too much and just gives you a reason to get stressed. For example, when I was having ultrasounds every day for a week during my last FET. My body was changing so much every day. A normal woman wouldn't have a clue what was going on and wouldn't be subjected to all of that stress. I have friends that have had a very low first pregnancy beta number. They go through hell for two days as they wait for the second number to see if it doubles (yes, they are pregnant) or if it falls (No, they are not). All of this takes place before a woman would normally even take a home pregnancy test.

The bottom line is that Eric and I chose to go down the fork on the road of fertility treatments and all that entails. We accepted that we had a responsibility to every embryo, that we made the choice to proactively create. Granted God was ultimately the creator of every one of them, but we certainly put our hands in the process. We had the responsibility to obey God and not leave any of them behind.

The process of the FETs with our totsicles surpassed my every expectation of how difficult and painful it would be. That is, unfortunately, part of that fork on the road that we chose. Sometimes you have a relatively smooth road like we did the first go around and sometimes it is incredibly rough like our second trip down the road.

I do not share any of this to discourage fertility treatments. As I said, I firmly believe that this was the fork on the road that God wanted us to take. <u>I would not change one thing we did</u>. I can say that in confidence because every decision we made was absolutely bathed in prayer. There were times when Satan would try to make me think that we made a wrong choice, but God always reminded me that He was with me on that road. The peace that gives me is priceless. I strongly encourage you to pray about every decision you make. Whether you go to church every Sunday or have never said a prayer in your life, God will listen.

Circling Back Around

When I looked at the verse in Ecclesiastes recently that Devon shared with me that afternoon on the bridge, I looked at it with new eyes. Ecclesiastes 11:5 (NIV), "As you do not know the path of the wind, or how the body is formed in a mother's womb, so you cannot understand the work of God, the maker of all things." In the past I focused on the part in the middle about the body being formed in the mother's womb. Perhaps that was false hope, but it was the hope I needed just to get through that time and I am grateful. Today that verse reveals this truth: I may not understand the path. The path of my infertility or the path of my life, but I know that God is working through it all. My experiences - successful fertility treatments, unsuccessful fertility treatments, miracle pregnancy, and high risk pregnancy - are all ways that I can relate to infertile women.

As I said, all of these things are so easy to say and understand after you have had the time to heal and process the whole journey of infertility. I have gained this perspective after a lot of tears, prayer, and introspection. I wish that when I was in the midst of my infertility struggle that I had the opportunity to talk to someone who had been through the same struggles. Someone who made it to the other side of Infertility Road and found a strength she never knew she had. A strength that she never would have had if she hadn't gone down that tough road.

My prayer is that some of it will speak to you. I hope it will help you take care of your precious heart while you are on your journey through infertility. Don't lose yourself while you are trying to become a mother. You may even find yourself in the process.

Chapter Nine – In Eric's Own Words

I am fortunate to be married to one of the most supportive husbands in the whole world. Not only does my very private husband support my desire to write *our* story so that I can help people, but he wanted to be a part of it. When I first started writing he came to me and asked if he could contribute and write something for the book. Knock me over with a feather. My husband, who by his own admission has read only one book – my book – in the last twenty years. My husband whose writing is limited to texts with his friends and emails at work. And now he wants to write something for me. For *you*.

I will be honest, ladies. Getting to read his thoughts was worth writing this book all on its own. Eric is a man of few words. But you better believe that his few words are carefully thought out and worth their weight in gold…

"I'm not going to lie. If it were left up to me we would probably only be somewhere between chapter 4 and chapter 5 of this book in our lives right now. You see, I can always push off until tomorrow what can be done today. I'm sure Stephanie would tell you that I can push off until next month what needed to have been done last week. Thank God for His divine nudges that for me often come from the look on Stephanie's face to say, "Yes, we should go talk to a reproductive endocrinologist" or "Yes, I think going to a counseling session with another couple will be very beneficial" and especially, "Yes, let's thaw out those totsicles and try for a few more kids." Anyone who knows me knows that I am "quiet", "laid back", "easy going", "nonchalant", "witty", or as some may say, "non-communicative", "procrastinator", "non-committal", "smart ass", or even "lazy". All of these are true to a degree which is why going through something that is as serious, emotional, schedule-driven, and time consuming as infertility was and is very difficult to internalize. And when you have the personality that I do, all you do is internalize, or ignore, some of the reality going on around you. Don't get me wrong. I was invested in the process we were going through but I believed it was my job to be the level head, the rock, and to show no emotion. In the next few paragraphs, hopefully I can give a glimpse into what infertility is like for the Y chromosome.

Check Your Pride at the Door

Check your pride at the door. This is the first thing I would say to any man who is facing infertility in his life. You can't fix everything and you can't do it all on your own. If you could, we wouldn't be having this conversation in the first place. My reality check came when after multiple tests, ultrasounds, and drug trials for Stephanie, I heard the words, "We should have Eric tested as well." Of course I'm thinking, "OK, so I need to have a blood test and maybe a urine test? They said they needed a sample. What other samples are there? Oh, you want a sperm sample?!?" That is when I learned checking my pride would not be enough. I needed to swallow it whole. Only men who have gone through infertility know what "the walk of shame" truly is. No, it's not a co-ed leaving a frat house at 10am Sunday morning to walk back to her dorm. It's actually middle-aged men being summoned by a 25 year old nurse, handed a cup, and shoved in a room with a leather chair. With my pride now firmly in the pit of my stomach, we waited for the results. Count, check, and double check. Motility (new word for me) was much like my personality. Next was the ultrasound which I still sometimes have nightmares about. No, there was no pain. Only extreme embarrassment and humiliation. I've never talked about how much of a shock to my system the initial testing was, partly because I don't "communicate" but more so because what I had to go through physically throughout the entire process was a mere drop in the bucket compared to what Stephanie or any female goes through during fertility treatments. I tried to keep a smile on my face any time I had to make the "walk of shame" (although not too big of a smile because that may give off the wrong impression to the nurse or other men waiting with their heads hung). It was the least I could do.

Another example of needing to check your pride is that other guys have NO IDEA what infertility is all about. I know I wouldn't have, nor would I have wanted to hear about it. We get the same comments and questions such as, "When are you guys going to have kids?" or "We need to have kids at the same time so they can play ball together!" or "At least you know your boys can swim." Ok, I know that last one is a little out of place but let me explain. This is yet another situation you will run into if you are so lucky to have a successful fertility treatment and become pregnant - especially with twins. I can remember it like it was yesterday. We were at my ten year high school reunion and Stephanie was pregnant with Ethan and Ella. She left after about 30 minutes which left me to fraternize with all of the guys I had not seen in a while. While talking it up at the bar, one of my friends asked where Stephanie was and I said, "She's pregnant with twins and left early." The next thing out of his mouth? You guessed it: "Awesome! At least you know your boys can swim." The easy thing to do is just smile and chuckle but standing with other friends that knew the truth I replied, "Well, they can't, which is why we have twins." Talk about changing the subject fast. It happened repeatedly and it still happens today when I tell people about our family. "Wow, fertile bunch!" Usually I simply smile but occasionally I will get the nudge to go into our story. That individual probably is not impacted by infertility directly but I think by giving someone the perspective then just maybe they will be a little more prepared in the event it happens to them or to someone they know.

No Ladies, We Don't Understand

By the grace of God, we men are not born with the overload of hormones that make you ladies tick. In normal everyday life with no foreign chemicals involved, we can't understand what's going on in your heads. Now take those hormones, charge them with the emotions of infertility, and add a double shot of more chemically engineered hormones and we certainly don't understand. We physically, mentally, and emotionally *can't* understand. That does not mean we don't care; it simply means we have no idea how to help. And if other guys are like me, we shut down even more. We will listen - try to listen - but there were countless times that in my head I screamed, "I have no idea what I'm supposed to say to make you feel better!" It's times like these that we too feel helpless. We want to be able to say the perfect thing that will make you feel better. Often times we will say what we believe is sound advice or encouragement and even a "fix it" comment. It takes several failed attempts before we realize that there is no "fix it" comment that we can say. They don't exist. And yes, there will be times that we seem annoyed that you want to talk about it again (especially if there is a game on) and yes, some of those times we actually will be annoyed. I had to remind myself often that she needed to get it out in the open just so she knew that at least one other person heard what was going on in her mind and in her heart. Still, I usually did not understand why it was so upsetting or why one particular comment from someone or an image she saw would set off the emotions. But what I did come to realize is that the emotions were and are very real and very raw. So ladies please excuse us for not being as upset as you are or even recognizing and reacting to each time that you are truly upset and need us to identify with your struggles, especially when you need us to initiate a conversation. We simply do not get it. No matter how many times we see you in pain and listen to you pour out your emotions, odds are that we won't realize the next time you need us to share the burden. We will, however, always be willing to listen, be a shoulder to lean on, and awkwardly kiss you on the head and say, "sorry". Frankly, sometimes that's all we can do.

Along for the Ride

Secondary infertility: what does that mean? Either you are infertile and you don't have kids or you were infertile but now you have kids. Again, I'm simple minded. But really, what is "secondary infertility"? I always knew we would eventually have to deal with our frozen embryos and most likely that would mean a FET. I was also very capable of completely blocking that reality out of my mind while we were simply trying to survive with three toddlers at home. We would get the bill every February or March for the totcicles' annual rent. I would make the same obnoxious joke about it every year and then file it back into that special place in my brain that even I don't enter. Eventually time and an impatient spouse caught up to me and we realized that it was time to go down that secondary infertility road. I'll admit, I was excited. Certainly not about continuing on the journey of infertility treatments or about the thought of the additional cost of raising more kids, but I was excited because to me this was an easy, no pressure, softball toss to the man upstairs. Like I said before, in my mind we had already defeated infertility and had three healthy kids to show for it. Now all we needed to do was let God drive. Stephanie would be the co-pilot and I would lay in the back and enjoy to ride. I was really at peace with going through the treatments and coming out on the other side with anywhere from 4 to zero kids. If it was in His plans, we could handle it. Almost everyone that we talked with about going through a frozen embryo transfer had the same exact thought: if it works, great! If it doesn't, well then we still have three great kids at home. It was the ultimate win-win situation. If you have read this book up to this point, then you know that Stephanie did not share the same thought process. How could she? She wasn't just along for the ride. She was actually the mode of transportation.

It took a while for me to realize just how alone she felt and in fact, how alone she truly *was* in the midst of our "secondary infertility". Honestly I was not required to do anything other than be at the actual embryo transfer and that was only because she couldn't drive after having a

Valium. There was no sample needed from me, no "walk of shame" to make. So it was easy to let my natural personality of "que sera sera" shine through. It also made it difficult for me to understand the toll it took because frankly I wasn't really on this part of the journey. When we initially went through infertility I never missed an appointment, not even a blood test. In the second round I think I only made one appointment aside from the actual transfer. Not because I didn't care, but I wasn't needed. It wasn't new to us so no reason to take off work. And if I did take off, it was to take over childcare responsibilities. Ultimately I just wanted the second tour to be over and the outcome to be what it was going to be. Not realizing how much of a burden Stephanie was carrying during the year of our secondary infertility is probably where I failed the most in our journey.

It Ain't Over Til…Well, Never

Stephanie began this book talking about our ten-year journey with infertility. To me the word 'journey' means constant, ongoing, and often times a struggle. I honestly never thought about our situation as a "ten year journey". Sure, it was most definitely a journey and a struggle for me when we were in the midst of testing, IUIs, our first full IVF cycle, and certainly during the thirteen weeks in the hospital battling a high-risk pregnancy. But in my mind that journey ended on October 17, 2006. Infertility meant that we couldn't have a child. Well, two crying babies meant that we could and that infertility had been defeated in our lives. In simple male logic, we had won. In fact, we were blessed with two babies so we not only won but we kicked its ass. To us males, so much comes down to beginnings and endings, problems and solutions, wins and losses. But unfortunately this mindset is not unique to men. I believe this is a universal perspective that is shared by those that are never directly impacted by infertility. If you are successful with fertility treatments like we were, then it is certainly the sentiment shared by most. Even if you are not successful with your initial treatments, most people have the idea that there is always the next treatment and if that fails, then there is adoption. Either way, there is always a solution or fix to your problem. That was my exact thinking when we were in the midst of our initial infertility battle. The end goal was a child. God's timing was not going to be the same for everyone and for some His plans may not include a child at all but there was always the thought that there will be resolution. I still believe this to be true but what I have learned after many years is that the struggle with infertility will always be part of your life.

Chapter Ten – In Her Own Words

A couple of months after I started writing this book, I made a decision. I had been writing quietly and had shared my decision to write a book with a few people. As I began to write more, my passion to help as many women as possible grew. As my passion grew so did my excitement about the book. I was on fire about my project. I decided that it was time to share my mission with a wider audience – Facebook. I wrote a status update that basically outlined what I was doing and hit "share" before I could look back. When Eric got home I told him I did something that he probably wouldn't be crazy about. My private, anti-social-media husband laughed and just shook his head. As different as we are, he shares my passion for helping people, so he wasn't mad.

The reaction I got from my friends (and even friends of friends) was astounding. Everyone was so supportive. Friends who I wasn't even aware struggled with infertility sent me private messages and shared their story. They were so grateful that someone was willing to talk about the taboo subject of infertility. I read each and every story and was amazed by these women's strength. There was a wide variety of experiences and paths taken and so much wisdom gained from each of them. The other blessing that came from me sharing was being reconnected with Rachael. Rachael and her husband were in our infertility counseling sessions. Rachael also happens to be an editor and was excited to jump on the project with me. I was so grateful!

Rachael and I decided to include some of these ladies' insight and wisdom in my book. Everyone's journey through infertility is different. I hope that there have been times as you read about my journey that you felt a connection. I really think that some of these other women's stories will be a blessing to you, too. I appreciate each and every one of these women who were willing to share their stories in the hope that they could help someone else.

The Agony of Infertility

"We tried to conceive for over a year before I got pregnant. My first pregnancy ended in a miscarriage. The ER doctor stoically told me, "It was nature's way of taking care of things." I had to wait another three months before we could even try again. It was the longest three months of my life. All the waiting was so hard. I felt like I had no control over my own path. Everything was out of my hands. After the three months, I immediately got pregnant but suffered my second miscarriage on my birthday. It was then that I got mad. I was angry with God. Why was I suffering like this? I did everything I was supposed to do. I was good. I waited until I got married. Why can't I have the one thing in the world I want?"

Amelia

"Saturday was my 55th birthday and it would have been nice to have family to help "celebrate". One of my friends was out of town to be with her daughter who just delivered her first baby and another friend was busy moving her daughter back to college. I was reminded how our friendship had changed when she was a new mother with this girl and I was trying desperately to conceive. I tried not to think how sad it made me to know that at this season in my life I would never be moving a child to college or be a grandmother. I almost made plans for a "pity party, table for one". I remember being bitter, angry, crying and upset with God. I even prayed for a special needs baby. Anything. I remember the monthly emotional rollercoaster ride of hoping followed by the feeling of failure."

Monica

Full Heart Empty Womb

"One of the hardest parts was when people asked, "When are y'all going to start having kids?" or, "You better start having them now because you are not getting any younger!" After four miscarriages, I wanted to tell people that it wasn't for lack of trying, but instead I put on a brave face and just said, "God willing, hopefully one of these days." Another hard part was not knowing what was wrong with me. Why could everyone get pregnant and have babies when I just got pregnant and ended up losing them all? Was God mad at me? Did I do something wrong to cause this? Was it my fault?"

Ashley

"One of the hardest parts was living in two week increments. Two weeks to ovulate, two weeks to see if it worked. The constant rise and fall of hope and hurt was sometimes too much. Even when I knew I needed to step back and gain some balance, my mind said, "What if this is the month?" You get so far down the journey it is really hard to stop. Luckily for me, it did work in the long run."

Christy

"After ten months of trying to get pregnant, I finally saw the words "you're pregnant". I couldn't believe my eyes. My excitement was short lived. At my fist appointment everything seemed great. However, my first ultrasound at 8 weeks showed that our baby didn't have a heartbeat. It was a long two weeks between when we found out and when the D & C was scheduled. We moved to Jacksonville, FL from Nashville immediately afterwards for my husband's job. He traveled all the time, I didn't know anyone, and didn't have a baby. I was miserable, felt fat, and my face had acne for the first time in my life due to hormone issues."

Casey

"My husband and I both wanted children but were never able to have them. I had a laparoscopy and discovered that both of my tubes were blocked. The only way to conceive was through IVF but unfortunately we didn't have that kind of money. In 2009 we divorced. I guess you could say that infertility was a major strain in our marriage. A few years later the doctors discovered a tumor that totally engulfed everything. I had to have a total hysterectomy which shattered all hope that was left."

Amy

"Whether you deal with infertility for two, five, or ten years, all the questions and feelings of inadequacy are there. You never know when or if you will get pregnant. For some it is a relatively easy fix. For others it is long, drawn out, and invasive. We all have the same feelings. You feel inadequate. Broken. You ask, "Why can't my body do the most basic thing that a woman's body should do? Will I ever be a mom? Will I be forced to grow old and not leave anything of myself behind - a testament to the love that I have for my wonderful husband?""

Patterson

"Infertility is horrible. No easy way to spin it, it is the pits. For whatever reason, God put my husband and me on that path. We did actually get pregnant four times, though all were chemical pregnancies. That is another curse of infertility. Many women have chemical pregnancies and have no clue, they just think their period is a little late. When you are getting blood tests at exactly two weeks later you not only know what has happened but then you experience the grief of what has happened. Not to mention my body would not completely allow the pregnancy to end. I would have to get mini D&Cs in the office to get my levels back to zero. Ironic that I couldn't maintain a pregnancy but also that I couldn't rid myself of one either!"

Nancy

"I tried to go to counseling. She did nothing but try to convince me I was fine without a baby, when that was the only thing I felt would "cure" me. Also, I don't think she was a Christian, because when I spoke of my faith in God and how I asked for His guidance, she once asked about "my" god. In other words, she didn't appear to share my views that He is the only God. And that with HIM I felt all things were possible. I truly believed that God wouldn't give me such desire for a child if He didn't have plans for me to have it. And I was open to adoption, but just wasn't emotionally ready for that yet. I was emotionally drained after three failed attempts (my second time around)."

Robyn

"My sister and I were both going through fertility treatments at the same time. My mom had a very hard time with it. Moms fix things and this was something she couldn't fix. She listened to us cry and tell her about our struggles and she felt powerless."

Amelia

"I don't have the anger or bitterness anymore when I hear that someone else is pregnant. It's not that in the past I didn't want them to be pregnant. It just made my heart *ache* so much."

Jill D

Which Fork on Infertility Road?

"After four years, numerous tests, several rounds of Clomid®, two failed IUI attempts, many tears shed, and many nights and days being angry, my husband and I decided to try IVF and all that goes with it. On our first attempt I got pregnant with twins. Writing that makes it seem so easy but as everyone with infertility knows, there is nothing easy about it. I cried every time a co-worker, relative or friend got pregnant. I cried when they asked me to prosecute the child abuse cases in my office because how could people abuse their children when all I wanted so desperately was to have one? I cried every time someone would ask me, "So are you next to get pregnant?" or, "When are you going to start having babies?" I wondered that exact thing daily."

Jill S.

Full Heart Empty Womb

"It felt like forever before we could even test to see what was going on. We knew something was wrong but we had to wait until we hit the magical 12-month mark. My husband had his sperm tested. He beamed when we got the voicemail with his favorable results. "Really good sperm here, excellent specimen!" So, I guess it is all *me*. After testing we discovered that my hormones were low. I got a prescription for a hormone and we were *ordered* to have sex every other day. I like sex as much as the next person but having a set schedule is no easy feat! I was tired, feeling wacky from additional hormones, and resentful I had to go to these lengths in the first place. This is when a supportive husband really helps. Flowers, back or foot rubs, anything to relax and achieve "the mood"! We persevered and after three months we had our good news and a positive pregnancy test!"

Patterson

"Infertility is something that is hard for me to accept because I never considered myself infertile. Actually, I considered myself to be VERY fertile. I could get pregnant really easily, but I just could not stay pregnant. I later learned that not being able to carry a baby to full term is considered infertile. So I guess I fit that bill - four times over. My path is different than some that aren't able to get pregnant. But I still feel your pain. I had four different miscarriages with four different diagnoses. None of them were related. So even though I was able to get pregnant, in the end I still had no baby."

Ashley

"This is both my husband's and my second marriage. Mine was what gets affectionately called a "starter marriage". His was much longer and resulted in two sons, after which he had a vasectomy. Fast forward ten years, we were by then married and ready to start figuring out how to have our own kids. We checked into vasectomy reversals and they were pretty expensive for us and not foolproof. We decided to check into sperm donors and it turns out it was MUCH cheaper. Luckily for me, my husband knew that sperm was the least of the things that make a father (while still incredibly important!). So on to check donor profiles and get started. Little did our little naive hearts know, but I couldn't get pregnant."

Christy

"Several months after my miscarriage we decided to visit a fertility clinic because I could not get pregnant again. I knew in my heart that day that I would have a baby. I wasn't sure what I would have to do but I just knew I would someday have a baby of my own. I believe with my whole heart that God spoke to me that day and told me to follow the process and trust my doctor. That is what we did. We found out that my husband has a morphology problem with his sperm. We were not defeated. In fact, we felt completely the opposite. "Yay!" we thought. We have a problem. We were almost elated to hear the words, "You are not getting pregnant on your own, but you can get pregnant with help." Skies seemed bluer. Life seemed happier and things were going to fall in to place for us. I had this calm feeling that I know came straight from heaven. I went through all the shots and all the terrible things that go along with harvesting the eggs. I didn't think twice. Every needle I put in my hip just made me giddy for the fact that the pain was taking me closer to having a baby."

Casey

Full Heart Empty Womb

"There are some people who don't believe in fertility treatments and think you should just accept if you can't have children. Until you are in that situation, I'm just not sure you can understand the unfulfilled desire and the devastation of wanting a child and not being able to have one. And multiple fertility treatments are not only exhausting, they are expensive. Trying to justify the decision to try again versus living with the continued desire (and not being able to have a child) is such a difficult choice to have to make."

Robyn

"Denial. That is the fork in Infertility Road that I decided to take. I had no problems getting pregnant with my first child. We have been trying to get pregnant again with no success after three years now. Now I know that I have what is known as Secondary Infertility. I know I could get some more tests done but I was able to get pregnant before. What is wrong with me now? How has my body changed so much?"

Jill D

"They unfortunately never found out exactly why I could not have children. The thought is that my hormone receptors were off balance but there is no good way to test for it or even fix it. We did look into surrogacy, but the option is extremely expensive. Trust me, infertility is expensive but this is a whole new ballpark expensive. We also went down the road of adoption. After several matches that just weren't right, we decided that we aren't really cut out for that avenue either. I am sure many people can't understand wanting something so badly and then deciding to just stop before achieving that goal. But along the journey to try to add a child to our life we realized our life isn't that bad. Really it is pretty awesome! We are not missing anything, we just wanted to add to it. Honestly we are at peace that we tried all options and it just wasn't meant to be. I feel as if all things happen for a reason and I believe that we were put on our fertility journey to help us strengthen our love for each other, grow our marriage, and to count our blessings."

Nancy

What Helped Me Survive Infertility

"I read books on infertility. I did yoga and exercised. It helped me have another goal to aim for outside of getting pregnant. I chose to not discuss my infertility with many people. I really only shared with my parents, my husband, and two or three close friends while I was trying and going through fertility treatments. I had this fear of people knowing. Knowing that it was almost time to find out and knowing that it didn't work. Because I was afraid they would ask me about it when I wasn't ready to talk. I certainly wasn't ashamed of our infertility. I just wanted to talk about it when I felt strong enough to talk about it. And I didn't want others talking to one another behind my back and predicting the outcome based on my behavior. I don't mean this to come across as mean or catty. I just didn't want others dwelling on it like I was having to do, day in and day out."

Robyn

"At first, it was very lonely. I didn't want to tell anyone because I didn't want them to pity me or feel uncomfortable trying to find words to make me feel better – or worse, think there is something wrong with me. The first few miscarriages I kept to myself and tried to fix my heart on my own. I soon learned that the best medicine was to have support from others who could take some of your burden and pray for you when you couldn't find the words to pray for yourself. I had a wonderful group of women from my Sunday school class that formed a 'book club'. Without the love, support, and prayers of these women, I don't think I could have been as strong as I was."

Ashley

"I had a close group of family and friends that I emailed with updates on procedures and failures and ultimately success. They sincerely kept me motivated and cared for, but also gave me an outlet for my fears and frustrations."

Christy

"I felt a huge sense of relief once we decided to share our struggles with infertility with our Sunday school class. I was so angry with God about our situation so I couldn't be on my knees in prayer to Him like I should have been. I depended on my friends to say the prayers that I couldn't get out."

Amelia

"Some of my favorite phrases that I said to myself during treatment were, "God gives you what you need, not what you want" and the

Serenity prayer: "God grant me the serenity to accept the things I cannot change, the courage to change the things I can, and the wisdom to know the difference." They comforted me to know that as much of a control freak that I am, I really had no control over the situation and to just let God take the lead."

Nancy

Lessons Learned

"Throughout all of this, my faith was tested. I knew that God had a bigger plan and that it would work when His timing was right, but man some days it was hard to remember. He put my husband in a job working with men who had wives also going through the same fertility issues (Eric, and Windy's husband) for which I am so thankful. It is often overlooked how stressful this journey is on dads-to-be and I am so glad he had that network to talk to about our struggle and triumphs. One day after a disheartening report from the doctor, he came home and said, "Eric asked me how things were going and reminded me that this will all happen in God's time and we will be able to look back one day when we have a baby and see why timing wasn't right with each negative test or result." That was so true. And I often remember that day and apply that to other things in life. Thanks, Eric, who probably doesn't even remember saying it! When Maggie finally was born, we were financially in a better place so I could stay home with her, my husband was in a job that didn't have a busy season so he could be home more, we were in a house close to both sets of parents, etc, etc. It just made sense. I was thrilled to help my best friend decorate a nursery weeks after I experienced a failed IVF, and thrilled to help a friend with PPD take care of her newborn after another failed IVF. All things I couldn't have done if my timing had worked. I grew and learned from their experiences as new or expecting moms, lessons I am so grateful for."

Jennifer

"Make your private journey with infertility known to your close friends and church family and actively enlist their regular and furtive prayer support for God's blessing in this area of your life."

Windy

"Through the tears, struggles, and anger I grew closer to my husband and I knew in my heart that I would one day be a mom. I just wasn't sure how. My husband and I joke (now) that God waited to let us be parents because he knew we were going to have twins and we needed much more time to prepare. Since the twins, we have had another baby, Carson. We call him our frozen triplet as he was one of our frozen embryos. I can't imagine my life without these three boys. The wonder of, "Am I ever going to get to be a mom?" is over but the struggles still continue. I would love to be able to easily get pregnant and have another baby, maybe a girl this time. But again, we all know there is nothing easy about getting pregnant when you struggle with infertility. So instead I thank God daily for my three little miracle babies and that He chose me to be their mommy."

Jill S

"When I started to feel comfortable talking to more people about my situation, I realized there were so many women out there going through the same thing and suffering in silence. I soon became the one that people came to when it happened to them and they just needed someone to relate to what they were going through. My journey has made me more sensitive when I meet women because you never know what battles they are fighting."

Ashley

"Looking back, my fertility journey was not just a winding road, but a full on detour through crazy town in a clown car. There were moments when I dealt with emotions I never knew existed and there were experiences I would like to one day forget. There were times when I did not even recognize myself and there were times when I learned what I was truly made of. I gained a genuine sensitivity to others and learned how to give grace to those who unknowingly said really stupid things. I learned that I am a lot stronger than I ever thought I was and I came to the realization that going for an annual pap smear is really no big deal."

Sindy

"I broke down and prayed to God and said all the things that I had bottled up inside for so long. It wasn't fair. Why was this happening to me? Then I felt God say to me that life isn't fair. If life were fair then Jesus never would have died on the cross for my sins. I would never be able to spend eternity with Him in Heaven. Satan likes to remind me a lot about that period in my life. God continually reminds me that I am already forgiven."

Amelia

"Throughout my four miscarriages, I learned that life would go on and I could get through this. I learned that my body was not mine but God's and he had a plan he wanted to carry out, even if it was hard for me to go through at the time. God knew me better than I knew myself and, for whatever reason, He knew I wasn't ready. He also knew that I would have stopped after having a few children. If I had not had those miscarriages, I would never have met my precious baby boy we have today. The spunky, energetic, absolutely amazing miracle that God finally let me have would not be here today. Just one look at his breathtaking smile makes the pain I have been through worth it. "

Ashley

"My biggest advice for someone going through infertility is don't lose yourself in it. I spent many hours agonizing over planning things around treatments and medication times. I did finally realize a needle, syringe, and medicine can be taken with you. I laugh at some of the places I had my husband give me injections (like the corridor of Neyland stadium with 100,000 of my closest friends). Then I really got smart and realized I didn't even need him to give me the shot and that I could do it myself! Talk about freedom. We continued to take trips and spend money on other things and I am so glad we did. I could have probably had the most amazing European vacation on the money we did spend towards treatment but who's counting!"

Nancy

Other Thoughts...

"Just as we began to discuss starting a family, I was diagnosed with Multiple Sclerosis. At my neurologist's urging, my husband and I tabled plans to start a family until we had an idea of how the disease would progress. Two years later, I at 34 and my husband at 37, we once again sought to begin a family. This time our plans were sidetracked by my diagnosis with endometriosis. The doctors told us that pregnancy was highly unlikely. With an unquenchable desire to start a family, we started with two rounds of intrauterine insemination. When that was not successful, we started the invitro fertilization process. Our first attempt resulted in a miscarriage at 12 weeks, perhaps the most devastating period of my life. We tried again soon thereafter and were again unsuccessful. We tried one final IVF cycle. This time, we enlisted the prayer support of an elderly couple, the Dysons, and our friends and coworkers. The Dysons committed to pray for us each morning. The cycle was filled with disappointment after disappointment. The doctors told us it was extremely unlikely that we would be successful in getting pregnant. Nevertheless, we prayed unceasingly and the Dysons continued to pray for us. Against all odds and to the surprise of the medical community, I got pregnant with a precious little girl. I delivered our daughter, Ashlinn, on February 26, 2010 - five years to the day after I received my diagnosis of Multiple Sclerosis."

Windy

"As strange as it sounds, I always knew – always – that I would have trouble getting pregnant. It was just a gut feeling I had even as a teen. And the first time I ever heard about IVF I immediately thought, "That will be my path." At my insistence we started trying early in our marriage. After nine months of trying to conceive, we had our first appointment at our fertility clinic. Our first step was Clomid®. After my first round of IUI, I had a positive pregnancy blood test. Sadly that ended in miscarriage. We continued to try to get pregnant for a year before we decided to take a break. We were still young and technically newlyweds and all the pressure and stress was too much. About a year later we started again. We then had 3 unsuccessful IUIs. We met with our reproductive endocrinologist and decided to pursue IVF. Our first two rounds of IVF did not work. On our third round, I got pregnant but it ended in another miscarriage. We met with our RE who said, "You will be pregnant in the next year. We are so close and physically there is no explanation for you not to be pregnant. We just have to keep trying month after month like typical reproduction." I almost cried when she said that. For her to be so point blank and give me that hope, I knew she was sincere. I underwent a detailed blood work evaluation while simultaneously planning for another transfer in February 2010. The blood work revealed a genetic marker for a clotting disorder as well a few other things. We added baby aspirin and a prescription folic acid supplement to my daily medicine cocktail. In my 4th IVF cycle, we transferred three embryos. Two weeks later we had the long awaited positive pregnancy test! We had an ultrasound and saw that it was one baby, our sweet and precious Maggie. About two weeks later we had a scare when I had some spotting but we were so relieved to see that sweet heartbeat again. My husband almost fainted when he saw it. Typical pregnancy, minus an emergency cerclage at 20 weeks, and Margaret Anderson was born on October 25, 2010 after my water broke at the post office. In November 2011 right after Maggie's first birthday we went back to retrieve our remaining embryos. February 1, 2012 we transferred the two remaining embryos and on February 13, 2012 we learned I was pregnant. In subsequent blood tests my numbers didn't double or triple like they should have, so for almost a month until mid-March 2012 we were unsure if it was a tubal pregnancy or viable at all. Again, it was such relief to see that sweet single heartbeat on that ultrasound monitor. I had a preventive cerclage at 14 weeks, then a typical pregnancy until our big buddy, Henry, was born on October 17. So, technically I guess my babies are twins; they were conceived on the same day in the same lab and frozen (Maggie for a year, Henry for three), just thawed and implanted at different times."

Jennifer

Full Heart Empty Womb

"Will and I were married in '99 and I had two miscarriages in the first year after we were married (one while he was out at sea on the submarine). I was obviously devastated, but I knew we'd have a baby sooner or later. We kept trying and after those two initial pregnancies, there was nothing. We went to various doctors and specialists to have tests. They all agreed that I couldn't get pregnant. Will and I started researching adoption options. One day I had to see my doctor after I had a period that was horrible and unusually painful. She did a pelvic exam and she felt a mass. I was sent to the hospital immediately for contrast testing and ultrasound. They found a 10 cm dermoid cyst on my ovary. When they removed the cyst they had to remove 3/4 of my ovary. They also discovered that I had a moderate case of endometriosis. Will and I continued meeting with our adoption counselor in order to make some decisions about how we wanted to proceed. About 18 months after my surgery, I was on my way to the adoption agency to turn in our money order to start the process. I decided to make a stop at Kroger on the way to get a pregnancy test. My periods were never really regular and I was often late, but for some reason this time I decided to get a pregnancy test. I took that test in the bathroom of Kroger and got a positive! I was so excited I drove straight to Will's office to tell him. My pregnancy was really difficult and I spent a lot of time running back and forth to the ER because I was convinced I was going to have another miscarriage. Once I got past 25 weeks, I relaxed a bit but Noah never moved much where I could feel him in utero so I always panicked that something had gone wrong. After I had him, he was our miracle baby and I never expected I'd ever have any more children the natural way. Finding out I was pregnant with Jacson was an absolute shock to me! And now four kids later, I guess you could say that everything is okay in that department."

Brandi

Words of Encouragement

"After months without a cycle at all, I finally got a diagnosis of PCOS. January of 2008 was my lowest point. I was on a high dosage of a medicine that made me very sick to my stomach all the time. I'd wrapped up a project at work I was very involved with. And I knew my two closest cousins were both expecting babies in the next 8 months.

The morning yet another cousin sent a message to say she was pregnant saw me dissolved into tears. I couldn't imagine being left out of this circle of parenthood. How long would it be before I could join? What if it never happened?

One day in February, I sat at my desk and verified Scripture references. I did copy editing for adult Bible studies and checking that the authors put in the correct reference was part of my job.

I mistyped a reference, realizing it almost instantly, but here is what came up:

"He settles the barren woman in her home as the happy mother of children. Praise the LORD." –Psalm 113:9

God spoke to me through a typo. I knew He hadn't forgotten about me then. What I didn't know was the tiny bundle of cells that was my daughter, my Libbie, was already there, and nestled inside me.

Today, this once-barren woman is the mother of three children! Praise the LORD!"

Jessie

"One day we were sitting in Sunday school and my friend, Jessie, came up to me and led me out into the hallway. She said she felt like she needed to pray for me. She prayed over me right there in the hallway.

It was exactly what I needed."

Amelia

"A few years after my divorce, God connected me with an amazing man who had lost his wife to cancer. He already had two grown kids. He had been praying for a woman who did not have any kids nor want any. We are perfect together and I truly believe he is God's gift to me. His daughter recently gave birth to a little girl. She lives close by so I am able to help with the baby while her mom goes to work. I am exactly where God intended me to be."

Amy

"Even though so many couples go through this, I think it is so easy to feel alone! However it turns out for you, it will be okay. Whether you get to celebrate in the end, or grieve what you thought would be, you are still valuable. You can be fulfilled. You might need help to get through the grief, but you can still be happy."

Christy

"Just having people be there to let me talk it out, cry over it, or just be still probably helped me the most. Unless you have been there, it is hard to tell someone how they 'should' be feeling and that everything will be ok. But to have people be my crutch on those days I didn't feel like walking helped me more than any words ever could because I knew those people left me and continued to pray for me harder than I prayed for myself."

Ashley

Full Heart Empty Womb

"This week I found out that four people are pregnant. It was just too much all at once. My friend that knew what I was going through just came up and gave me a hug. She knew I was hurting and didn't have to say a word."

Jill

"I have been able to talk to and help three other women since my battle began. All have healthy babies now. They are all people I didn't know very well before this but somehow knew of my struggle and sought advice or comfort and I am always glad to give it. I'm sad that it still has such a negative, "embarrassing" attitude around it. There's nothing to be ashamed of, this is the way God made certain people and thank goodness he made genius scientists who can figure out how to help people through it and to become parents."

Jennifer

"Though our journey did not end with a child it was not a wasted ride. My husband and I discovered a whole new love and appreciation for each other. After over four years of multiple procedures and countless money and time spent, we realized that if the journey ends with our family remaining a party of two, that life will be just fine. In fact, better than fine! We have been blessed beyond measure with good jobs, a beautiful new home, our health, special friends, and wonderful family. Who are we to feel as if we are owed one more thing? It puts life into perspective to cherish what you do have and live for that rather than to regret or agonize over what you think is missing."

Nancy

THE END

Acknowledgements

God blessed me with so many wonderful people who have helped me on my journey through infertility and writing this book. Dr. Christine Whitworth, Jordan Vaughan and the entire staff at Nashville Fertility Center for their outstanding care and constant encouragement. Dr. Mary Anne Blake for being the best OB a gal could ask for. You visited me every day I was in the hospital on bed rest. I looked forward to seeing your warm smile each morning. You gave me the strength to cross off another day on the calendar. My editor, Rachael Hamilton. I thank God that He brought you into my life so many years ago. You supported me as we battled infertility together and then again as I wrote this book. Your faith in me gave me the courage to pursue my passion. Ginger Baldwin. I appreciate you sharing your fabulous photography skills for the cover. More importantly, thank you for your friendship. You were a constant cheerleader and prayer warrior for me. Ashley Rickel. God knew what He was doing when he brought you into my life. What a sweet friendship we developed in such a short time. I appreciate your awesome creativity and helping with my book cover. Last but not least, I thank all the brave women who contributed to the "In Her Own Words" chapter. Your honesty will bless a woman who reads your words. Thank you for being brave and talking about something that is so difficult and painful.

About the Author

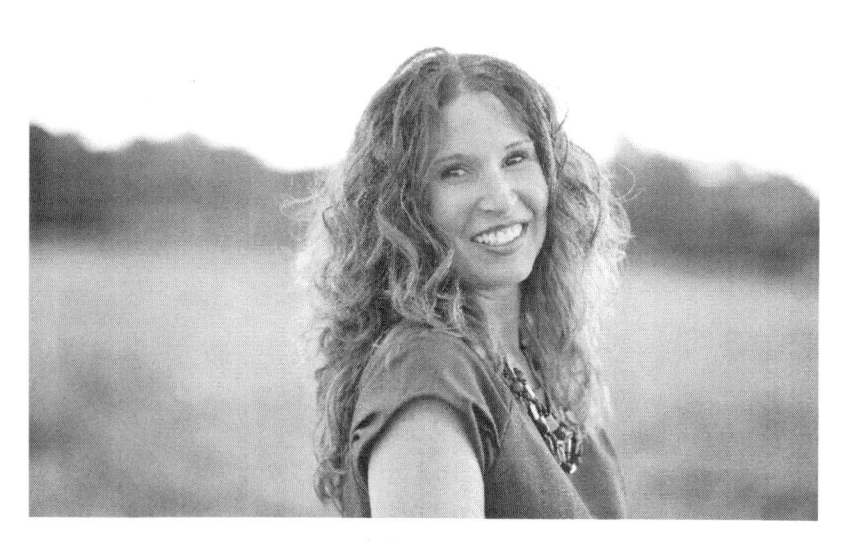

Stephanie is a native Texan that has spent the majority of her life at home in Tennessee. She is a true Southern girl who loves God, sweet tea, football and anything monogrammed. She married her college sweetheart, Eric, who taught her about true love and football. The "option" still stumps her because isn't there always an option to throw the ball?? After battling infertility for years, they were blessed with three children. In her first book, "Full Heart Empty Womb" Stephanie chronicles their journey through infertility and what she learned along the way. When Stephanie is not writing, she stays busy teaching preschool, volunteering, and caring for her family. If she is lucky, a hot bath and a good book are waiting at the end of a very full day. Stephanie is available for limited speaking engagements. You can follow her on her blog: fullheartemptywomb.blogspot.com and contact her at: fullheartemptywomb@gmail.com.